Principles & Procedures of
Nursing Foundations

(Advanced Nursing Procedures)

Includes All Important Procedures as per INC Syllabus

● Volume-II ●

Sushma Pandey MSc (MSN), DHA (Chennai)

Sujok Therapist
Associate Professor

KJ Somaiya School and College of Nursing
Sion, Mumbai, Maharashtra

Mohd. Atif Muzammil MSc (MSN)

Assistant Professor

KJ Somaiya School and College of Nursing
Sion, Mumbai, Maharashtra

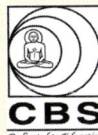

CBS
Dedicated to Education

CBS Publishers & Distributors Pvt Ltd

● New Delhi ● Bengaluru ● Chennai ● Kochi ● Kolkata ● Mumbai
● Hyderabad ● Nagpur ● Patna ● Pune ● Vijayawada

Principles & Procedures of Nursing Foundations

Volume-II

ISBN: 978-93-89261-87-5

Copyright © Publishers

First Edition: 2020

Published by **Satish Kumar Jain** and produced by **Varun Jain** for

CBS Publishers and Distributors Pvt Ltd

4819/XI Prahlad Street, 24 Ansari Road, Daryaganj, New Delhi 110 002, India.
Ph: 23289259, 23266861, 23266867   Website: www.cbspd.com
Fax: 011-23243014
e-mail: delhi@cbspd.com; cbspubs@airtelmail.in.
Corporate Office: 204 FIE, Industrial Area, Patparganj, Delhi 110 092
Ph: 4934 4934   Fax: 4934 4935
e-mail: bhupesharora@cbspd.com

Branches

- **Bengaluru:** Seema House 2975, 17th Cross, K.R. Road,
  Banasankari 2nd Stage, Bengaluru 560 070, Karnataka
  Ph: +91-80-26771678/79   Fax: +91-80-26771680
  e-mail: bangalore@cbspd.com

- **Chennai:** No. 7, Subbaraya Street, Shenoy Nagar, Chennai 600 030, Tamil Nadu
  Ph: +91-44-42032115   Fax: +91-44-42032115
  e-mail: chennai@cbspd.com

- **Kochi:** Ashana House, 39/1904, AM Thomas Road, Valanjambalam, Eranakulam 682 018, Kochi, Kerala
  Ph: +91-484-4059061-62-64-65   Fax: +91-484-4059065
  e-mail: kochi@cbspd.com

- **Kolkata:** No. 6/B, Ground Floor, Rameswar Shaw Road, Kolkata-700014 (West Bengal), India
  Ph: +91-33-2289-1126, 2289-1127
  e-mail: kolkata@cbspd.com

- **Mumbai:** 83-C, Dr E Moses Road, Worli, Mumbai-400018, Maharashtra
  Ph: +91-22-24902340/41   Fax: +91-22-24902342
  e-mail: mumbai@cbspd.com

Representatives

- Hyderabad   +91-9885175004
- Vijaywada   +91-74069-04007
- Patna   +91-9334159340
- Mangalore   +91-9741432102

Printed at: Magic International Pvt. Ltd. Greater Noida, UP, India

Contributors and Reviewers List

Contributors

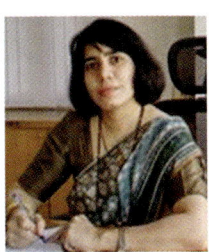

Avani Oke

Principal
KJ Somaiya School & College of
Nursing
Sion, Mumbai
Maharashtra

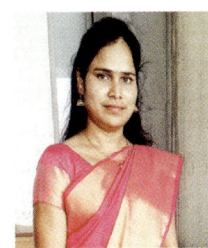

Swati Bhalerao

Assistant Professor
KJ Somaiya School & College of
Nursing
Sion, Mumbai
Maharashtra

Reviewers

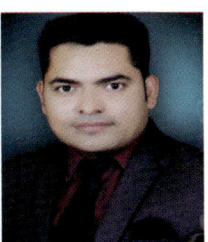

Farukh Khan

Principal
The Academy of Nursing
Sciences and Hospital
Gwalior, Madhya Pradesh

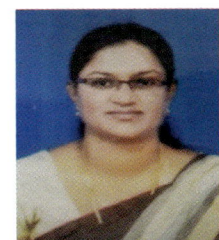

Rema Rajesh

In-charge Principal
Assistant Lecturer
Government College of Nursing
Durg, Chhattisgarh

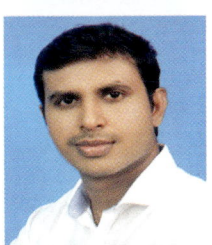

Manu KJ

Assistant Professor
Koyili College of Nursing
Kannur, Kerala

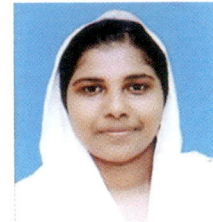

Shahina Afzal

Vice Principal
Azeezia College of Nursing
Meeyannoor, Kollam
Kerala

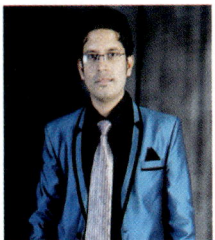

Mohammad Kashif Imran
MS General Surgery

Consultant
Sri Devaraj Urs Medical College
Kolar, Karnataka

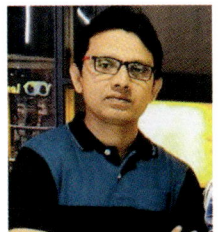

Shaikh Ismail

Assistant Professor
Hitech City College of Nursing
Gulbarga, Karnataka

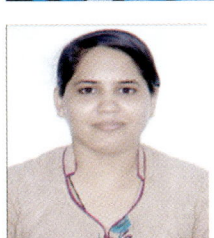

Ranjana Sandeep Paradkar

Associate Professor
Datta Meghe Institute of
Medical Sciences
Smt. Radhikabai Meghe
Memorial College of Nursing
Wardha, Maharashtra

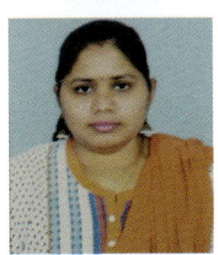

Veena Verma

Assistant Professor
Government College of Nursing
Raipur, Chhattisgarh

The names of the contributors and reviewers are arranged in an alphabetical order.

From Publisher's Desk

"Gaining knowledge is the first step to wisdom. Sharing it is the first step to humanity."

The above mentioned lines form the foundation stone of CBS Publishers and Distributors Pvt Ltd, the flag bearer in medical publishing. Headquartered in New Delhi, the national capital of India, CBS was established in the year 1972 and it has expanded its roots to grow as a pioneer in the field of medical publishing in Asia. CBS is one of the largest and the fastest growing publishers of medical books in Southeast Asia. We are partners in the education of undergraduate and postgraduate students for we believe in nurturing the brains of medicos since the beginning of their careers in medicine. CBS joins the hands with the medical students as their first choice since the very moment they enter the college with BD Chaurasia's Human Anatomy and CC Chatterjee's Human Physiology. CBS is the proud owner of many bestselling titles like OP Ghai's Textbook of Pediatrics, Manipal's Surgery, KD Chatterjee's Textbook of Parasitology, and the list goes on. CBS has successfully partnered in sculpting the careers of millions of medicos across the world.

Since establishment of "CBS Nursing Knowledge Tree", we have published many successful titles in the field of nursing and we have proved ourselves in the nursing fraternity in providing Quality Education.

Vision and Mission of CBS Nursing Knowledge Tree

CBS Nursing Knowledge Tree is conceptualized with a vision of being the first of its kind to bring the best quality books for education of Nurses. Keeping in mind the changing trends in the Nursing Education, we at CBS have taken up a mission to bring student-friendly and syllabus-based books written by Subject Experts from PAN India without compromising on the Quality of content and presenting it in a Unique manner.

Foundation Stones of CBS Nursing Knowledge Tree

- **Strong editorial support by the leading subject experts and faculties in Nursing from PAN India.** Every manuscript/proposal that is received is critically reviewed by our Editorial Board at various levels to ensure the Quality of content. A book is published only after all the parameters in our process management are satisfied.

- **Special care taken to publish Plagiarism-free matter.** With the copyright laws being highly strict these days, we at CBS are paying extra attention at various stages of publishing a book to crosscheck and avoid any copyright infringement.

- **Books authored by Subject Experts and Senior Faculties all over India.** Every title owned by CBS Nursing Knowledge Tree is written by the senior-most faculties and subject masters from every nook and corner of the country to provide them a bigger platform to share their knowledge and experience amongst budding nursing fraternity.

- **All the books developed as per INC syllabus and needs of the students without compromising on the Quality of the content.** Often students complain that some books are either not covering the complete syllabus or have too much content as compared to the syllabus. In this series, extra care is being taken to develop books strictly as per INC syllabus in the most student-friendly manner.

- **All books being reviewed by Top-notch faculties and Subject Experts to maintain high standards of Quality.** Every title goes through tough grilling regarding the content and the overall presentation by various top subject experts as reviewers. This ensures that only the Quality content gets published.

- **Best International standard layouts for every book.** Every title in CBS Nursing Knowledge Tree is designed and formatted in the best layouts of international standards because we strongly believe that every book deserves to be treated the Best!

- **Additional and Unique features given with every title.** Every title is accompanied by one or the other additional feature to complement the learning of students like—*Workbook, DVD, Last Minute Revision Notes*. We have also included many features like *How to make Most out of this Book, Assess Yourself* that contains questions and MCQs and other special boxes according to the need of the content.

Let's Join Our Hands Together

We can only bring the change that we want to see in Nursing Education with the support and cooperation of leading faculties in all Nursing specialties. If you envision the same, we are happy to welcome you to our panel of contributors and reviewers and let's take up this mission together of creating a Change in Nursing Education.

We crave cooperation from all the students and faculties to provide their genuine feedback on the quality of the books and how we can improve upon the deficiencies in future on the following email id: cbsvpdesk@yahoo.com. Constructive criticism with concrete suggestions for improvement for all our books will be highly appreciated.

Expanding Horizons

We are also highly active in attending various National Level Conferences and Meets organized by various Nursing Societies. We are keenly working to expand our horizons of associations by participating in conferences organized by **SOCHNI, ISPN, NRSI, ICMR, SOMI,** etc. every year. CBS has always been a forerunner and a big supporter of all National level Nursing Conferences. *If you have any National and State level conference proposals, we are happy to be the part of these conferences.*

Being Social is Our Aspiration

In this era of Social Media, we are happy being social as well by bringing you our Facebook page **facebook.com/ cbsnursingtree** of "CBS Nursing Knowledge Tree" to expand our reach to the maximum people in Nursing. It is a platform purely dedicated to bring the important aspects and latest updates and developments in various domains and fields of Nursing. It will be our privilege if you could connect with us and share your knowledge and experiences as well on our Facebook page.

I would like to invite all the readers to come and join us on our facebook page and share some input, information and literature.

With this vision and above features we are happy to announce the release of **Principles and Procedures of Nursing Foundations, Volume-II** by **Ms Sushma Pandey and Mohd. Atif Muzammil.**

Bhupesh Arora

Vice President-Publishing and Marketing

(NURSING Division)

CBS Publishers and Distributors (Delhi) Pvt. Ltd.

Email: bhupesharora@cbspd.com

Mobile: (+91) 9555590180

Foreword

It gives me an immense pleasure to write the foreword for the book "Principles and Procedures of Nursing Foundations, Volume-II", prepared by the two eminent teachers of KJ Somaiya School and College of Nursing.

The content of this procedure manual has detailed information to understand fundamental nursing procedures, which would benefit the pursuing students and graduates to maintain high standards of nursing practice.

The main purpose of this procedure manual is to prepare nurses to combine the highest level of scientific knowledge and skill with responsible, caring practice.

This manual will provide wide knowledge and fine nursing skills that can be transferred to the nursing students very effectively.

The manual has been designed by nursing teachers of the college in such a way that it reflects all the domains throughout the text, i.e. knowledge, development of attitude and skills. The preparation of nursing students by teachers starts with basic nursing procedures. These are strengthened over a period of time as advanced nursing procedures based on knowledge and skills.

A special feature of this manual is that it has been authored and contributed by experts with many illustrations and photographs, which would aid to reinforce the skills of nursing students.

The authors are confident that this book will prove to be a useful tool for undergraduate students as well as professional nurses working in different settings.

Avani Oke
Principal
KJ Somaiya School and College of Nursing
Sion, Mumbai, Maharashtra

Preface

This book "Principles and Procedures of Nursing Foundations, Volume-II", is a contemporary nursing practice book built upon the premise that nursing is both a caring and a knowledge-based profession. It has been designed to provide today's students with solid advance nursing principles to prepare them to meet the challenges of tomorrow. This cutting-edge text illustrates how to attain and integrate knowledge of theory and practice.

This book covers all the advanced nursing procedures which are used in medical and surgical nursing and instills an advance understanding of the procedures by the inclusion of proper procedural steps and their rationales. The procedures are explained in a systematic manner, emphasizing higher level of cognitive, affective and psychomotor skills needed to carry out the procedures. Each procedure has articles and their purposes along with their points to remember at the end, which will make them to understand and memorize the key concepts.

We are confident that not only nursing students and nurses will benefit from reading this procedure manual, but it will also provide a guideline for Nurse Educators for demonstrating procedures.

Sushma Pandey
Mohd. Atif Muzammil

Acknowledgments

We thank the **Lord Almighty** for giving us the strength and perseverance.

We are highly indebted to **Mrs Avani Oke**, Principal, KJ Somaiya School and College of Nursing for editing the procedure manual and also for her foreword.

We are thankful to **Ms Aswathy Aby, Associate Professor, DY Patil College of Nursing, Ms Priyadarshini John, Assistant Professor, DY Patil College of Nursing**, and **Ms Mini Nair, Chief Nursing Superintendent, KJ Somaiya Hospital and Research Center** for editing and providing professional assistance in developing this manual.

We extend our heartiest gratitude to the **Management and Faculty** of KJ Somaiya School and College of Nursing for supporting us. We appreciate the **Medical Surgical Department** for their professionalism toward the formulation of this manual.

Our special thanks to **Mr Satish Kumar Jain** (Chairman) and **Mr Varun Jain** (Managing Director), M/s CBS Publishers and Distributors Pvt Ltd for their wholehearted support in publication of this book. We have no words to describe the role, efforts, inputs and initiatives undertaken by **Mr Bhupesh Arora,** Vice-President (Publishing and Marketing), PGMEE and Nursing Division for helping and motivating us.

We would like to thank Dr Mrinalini Bakshi (Editorial Head and Content Strategist) for her editorial support on this project. We personally thank Ms Nitasha Arora (Production Head and Content Strategist), Dr Anju Dhir (Senior Scientific Coordinator/Editor), Mr Nitish K Dubey (Senior Editor) and all the production team members Mr Ashutosh Pathak, Mr Chaman Lal, Mr Phool Kumar, Mr Bunty Kashyap, Mr Prakash Gaur, Ms Tahira Parveen, Ms Babita Verma, Mr Chander, Ms Manorama, Mr Raju Sharma, Mr Vikram Chaudhary, Mr Manoj Chaudhary, Mr Manoj Malakar and Mr Arun Kumar for devoting laborious hours in designing and typesetting of the book.

Thank you all. Without you, this endeavor would not have been possible.

Contents

Chapter 1   Injections   1–3

Chapter 2   Administering an Intramuscular Injection   5–8

Chapter 3   Administering an Intradermal Injection   9–12

Chapter 4   Administering Subcutaneous Injection   13–16

Chapter 5   Intravenous Cannulation   17–20

Chapter 6   Intravenous Infusion   21–24

Chapter 7   Blood Transfusion   25–29

Chapter 8   Assisting in Surgical Scrubbing   31–34

Chapter 9   Assisting in Gowning and Masking   35–37

Chapter 10   Gloving   39–41

Chapter 11   Surgical or Wound Dressing   43–46

Chapter 12   Assisting in Removal of Sutures   47–52

Chapter 13   Oropharyngeal Suctioning   53–55

Chapter 14   Tracheostomy Care and Suctioning   57–59

Chapter 15   Monitoring Central Venous Pressure   61–63

Chapter 16   Assisting in Insertion of Central Venous Catheter   65–68

Chapter 17   Central Venous Catheter Care—Change Dressing   69–71

Chapter 18   Assisting in Thoracentesis   73–77

Chapter 19   Abdominal Paracentesis   79–83

Chapter 20   Care of the Patient with Chest Drainage   85–89

Chapter 21   Eye Irrigation   91–93

Chapter 22   Ear Irrigation   95–97

Chapter 23   Assisting in Endotracheal Tube Intubation   99–101

Chapter 24   Assisting with Obtaining a Pap Smear   103–106

Chapter 25   Assisting with Lumbar Puncture   107–110

Chapter 26   Assisting Patient with Continuous Ambulatory Peritoneal Dialysis   111–114

Chapter 27   Assisting with Insertion of Sengstaken-Blakemore Tube Balloon Tamponade   115–118

Chapter 28   Colostomy Care   119–123

Chapter 29   Intracranial Pressure Monitoring   125–128

Chapter 30   Cerebrospinal Fluid Flow Monitoring   129–130

Chapter 31   Pacemaker Implantation Procedure   131–137

Chapter 32   Assisting in Cardiac Catheterization   139–142

Chapter 33   Assisting in Application of Plaster Cast   143–147

Chapter 34   Skeletal Traction   149–152

Chapter 35   Skin Traction   153–158

Chapter 36   Assisting in Liver Biopsy   159–161

Chapter 37   Assisting with Bone Marrow Aspiration and Biopsy   163–166

Chapter 38   Assisting with Renal Biopsy   167–169

Chapter 39   Endoscopy   171–173

Chapter 40   Cystoscopy   175–177

Contents

Chapter 41	Proctoscopy	179–181
Chapter 42	Endoscopic Retrograde Cholangiopancreatography	183–185
Chapter 43	Colonoscopy	187–189
Chapter 44	X-ray	191–193
Chapter 45	Ultrasound (Sonography)	195–197
Chapter 46	Electrocardiogram (ECG)	199–201
Chapter 47	Electroencephalography (EEG)	203–205
Chapter 48	Stress Test	207–209
Chapter 49	Computed Tomography (CT)	211–213
Chapter 50	Magnetic Resonance Imaging (MRI)	215–217
Chapter 51	Barium Studies	219–220
Chapter 52	Barium Enema	221–222
Chapter 53	Intravenous Pyelography (IVP)	223–225
Chapter 54	Preparation and After Care for Mammography	227–228
Chapter 55	Initial Care of Patient in the Burn Unit	229–231
Chapter 56	Fluid Replacement in Acute Burns	233–234
Chapter 57	Range of Motion	235–236

Annexures

Annexure-I	*Fluid Calculation Chart*	*238*
Annexure-II	*Health Talk Assignment*	*239*
Annexure-III	*Medication Card*	*240*
Annexure-IV	*Braden Scale for Predicting Pressure Sore Risk*	*241–242*
Annexure-V	*VIP Score Visual Infusion Phlebitis Score (VIP Score)*	*243*

Contents

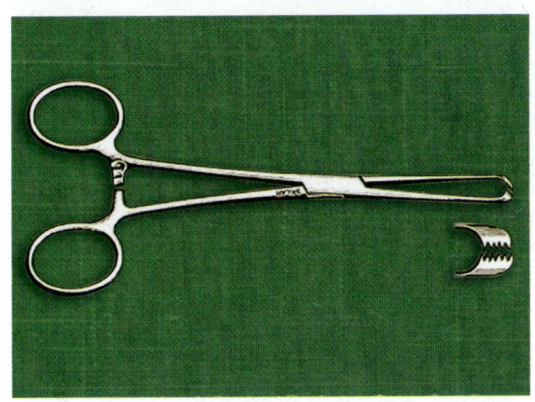

Allis forceps

Ambu bag

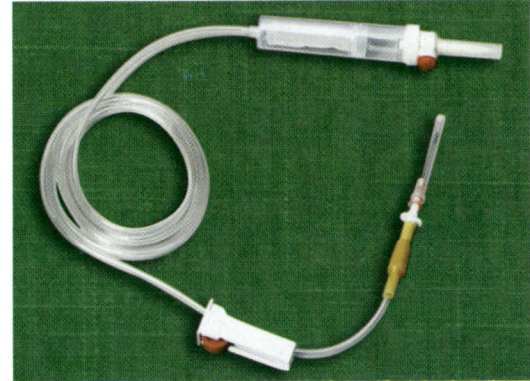
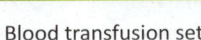

Blood transfusion set

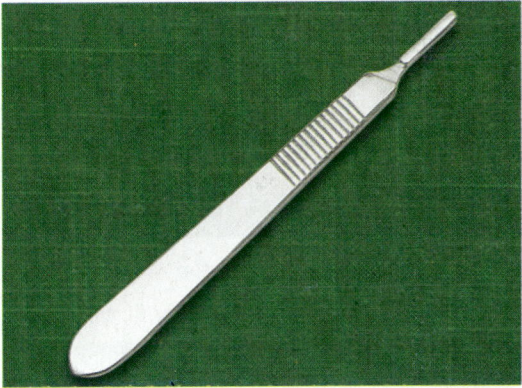

BP handle

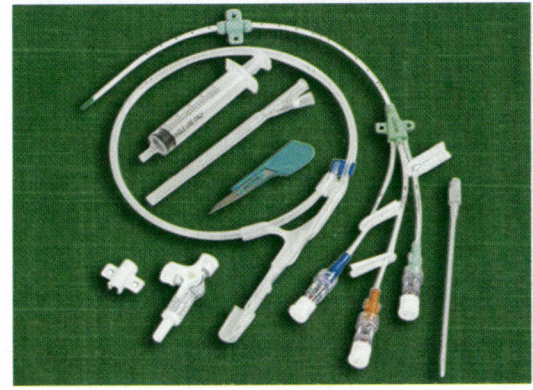

Central venous catheters

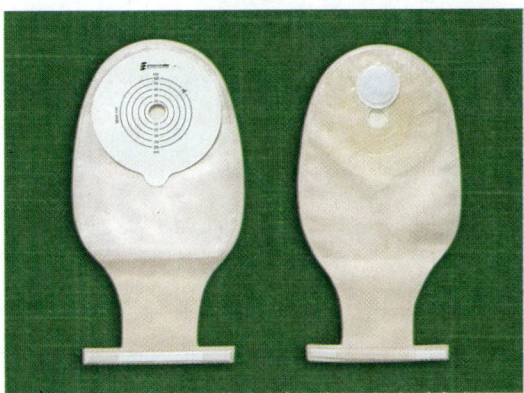

Colostomy bag

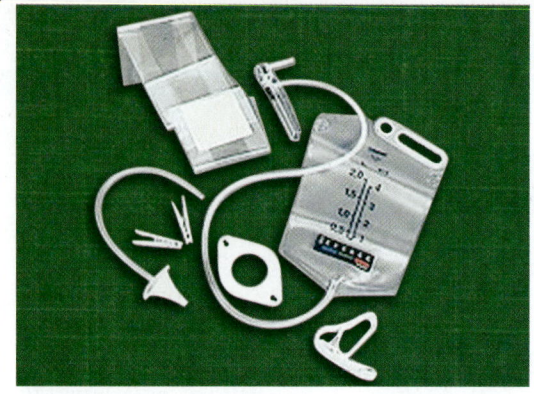

Colostomy irrigation kit

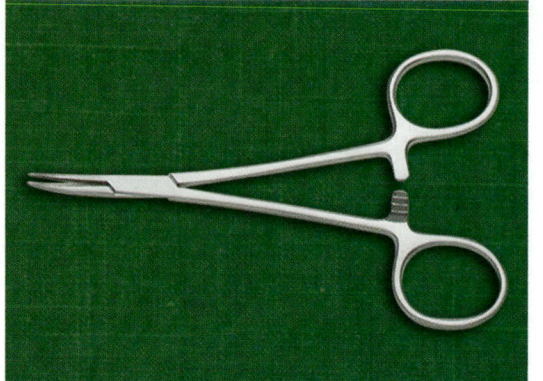

Curved mosquito forceps

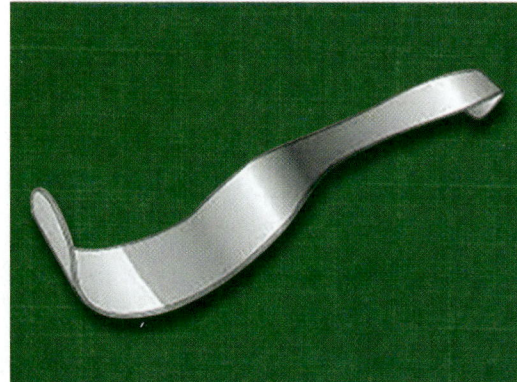

Deavers retractor

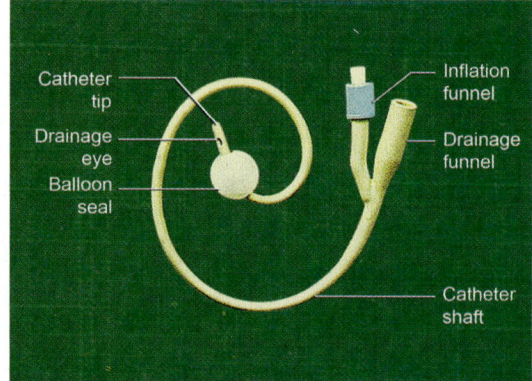

Catheter tip
Drainage eye
Balloon seal
Inflation funnel
Drainage funnel
Catheter shaft

Double lumen urinary catheter

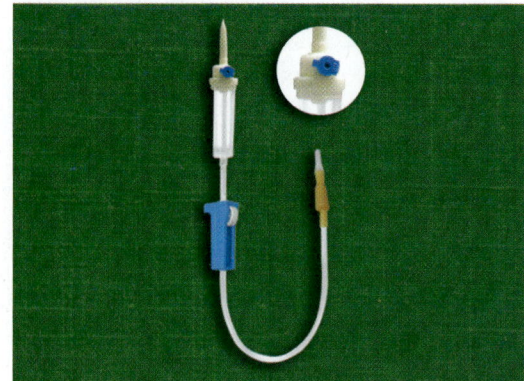

Infusion tubing

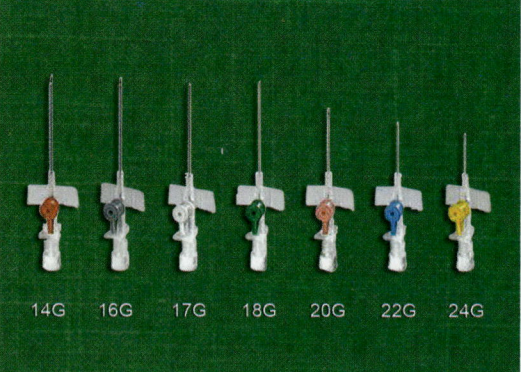

14G 16G 17G 18G 20G 22G 24G

IV cannula

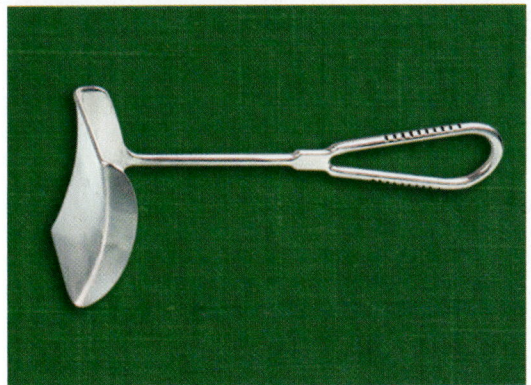

Morris-retractor

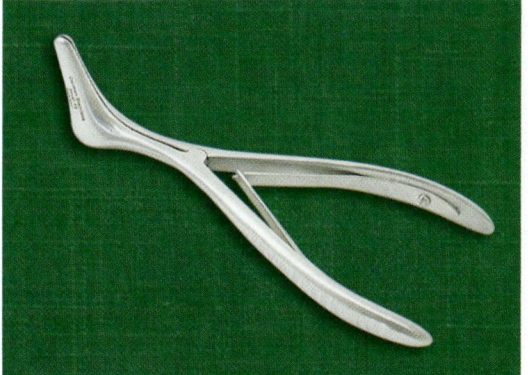

Nasal speculum

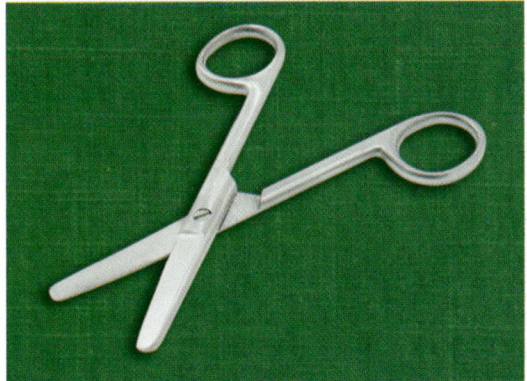

Stout scissors

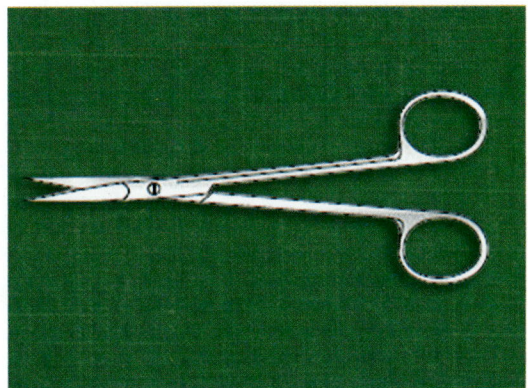

Stilly scissors

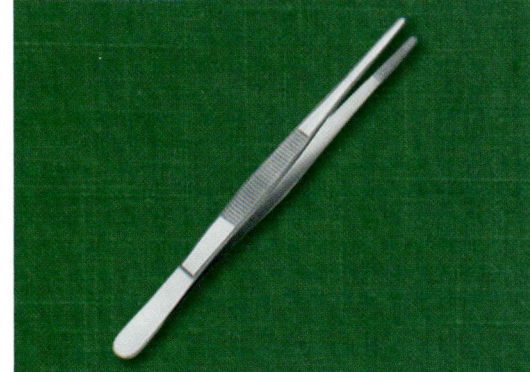

Thumb forceps

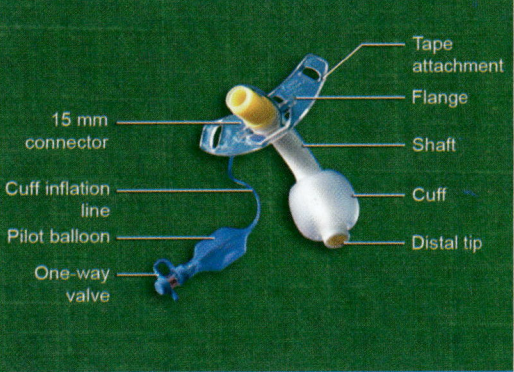

Tape attachment

Flange

15 mm connector

Shaft

Cuff inflation line

Cuff

Pilot balloon

Distal tip

One-way valve

Tracheostomy tube

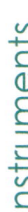

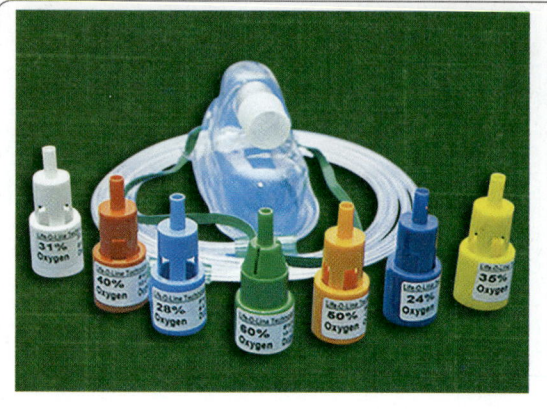

Venturi mask

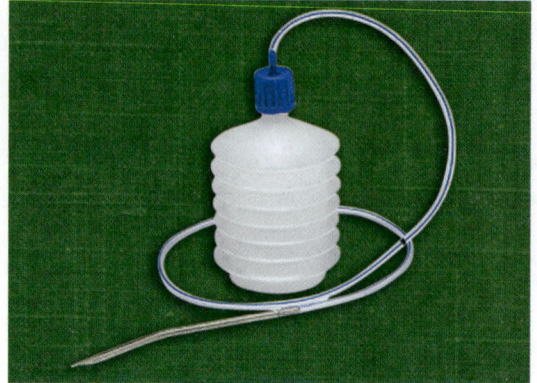

Wound drainer

Instruments

CHAPTER 1

Injections

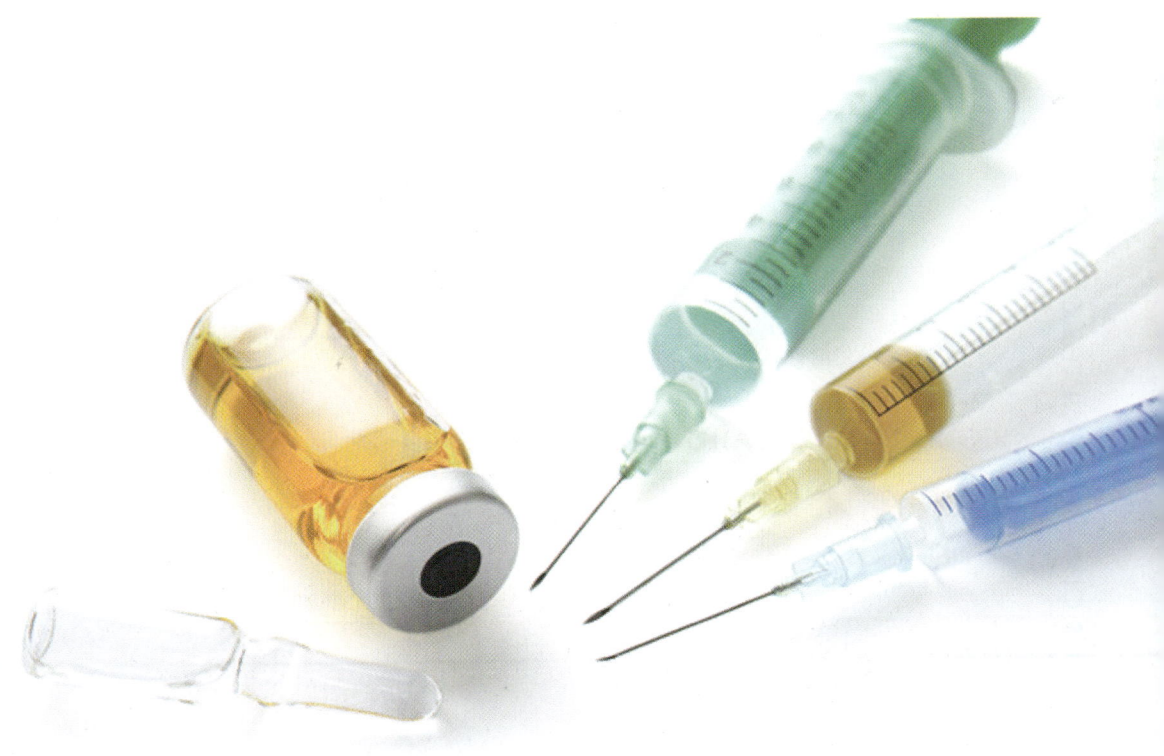

DEFINITION

Injection is the procedure in which a prescribed dose of medicine is injected through a syringe and needle into the body.

ROUTES OF DRUG ADMINISTRATION

- ❑ **Intramuscular:** Administration of medicine into deep muscle tissue.
- ❑ **Intradermal:** Administration of medicine into dermal layer of skin.
- ❑ **Subcutaneous:** Administration of medicine into subcutaneous tissue.
- ❑ **Intravenous:** Administration of medicine into a vein.
- ❑ **Intra-arterial:** Administration of medicine into an artery.
- ❑ **Intra-articular:** Administration of medicine into the joint space.
- ❑ **Intracardiac:** Administration of medicine into the heart.
- ❑ **Intraperitoneal:** Administration of medicine into the peritoneum.
- ❑ **Intrathecal:** Administration of medicine into the spine.
- ❑ **Intraocular:** Administration of medicine into the eye.
- ❑ **Intravaginal:** Administration of medicine into the vagina.

PARTS OF A SYRINGE (FIGS 1A AND B)

A syringe has three main parts: a barrel, a plunger and a needle. The barrel holds the medication. The plunger pushes the medication from the barrel through the needle. The needle delivers the medication into the injection site.

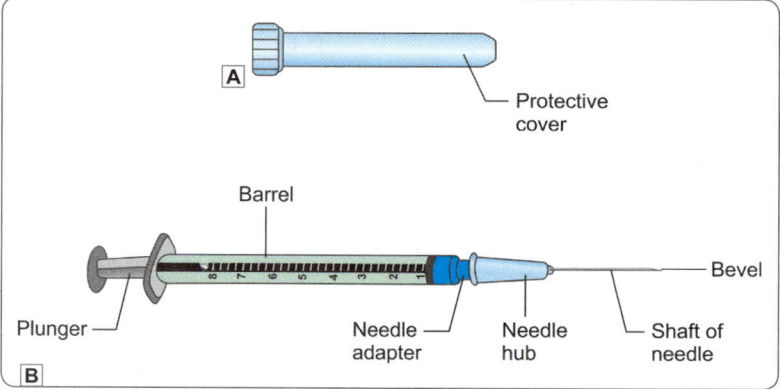

FIGS 1A AND B: Parts of syringe. **A.** Protective cover; **B.** Disposable syringe and needle (parts labeled)

RIGHTS OF MEDICATION ADMINISTRATION

- ❑ Right patient
- ❑ Right medication
- ❑ Right dose
- ❑ Right route
- ❑ Right time
- ❑ Right patient education
- ❑ Right documentation
- ❑ Right to refuse
- ❑ Right assessment
- ❑ Right to evaluation

SCIENTIFIC PRINCIPLES FOR INJECTIONS

Anatomy and Physiology

- ❑ The skin contains blood vessels and nerves. The common sites for injections are intramuscular, intradermal, subcutaneous and intravenous.
- ❑ Intramuscular injections are given on gluteal, deltoid, vastus lateralis and rectus femoris. There is well blood supply and poor supply of sensory nerves in these muscles.
- ❑ Subcutaneous injections are administer in loose alveolar tissues, which contains rich blood supply, lymph vessels and nerves.
- ❑ Intradermal injections are given at the inner aspects of forearm. Mostly given for local effects.

Microbiology

- ❑ Wash hands before and after the procedure to avoid cross infection.
- ❑ Use sterile syringe and needle for each patient.
- ❑ Use sterile water for dissolving drugs.
- ❑ Clean the top of vial with spirit swabs before inserting needle into the vial.
- ❑ Clean and discard the waste materials in appropriate container.
- ❑ The bacteria is always present over the skin, so clean the area of the injection to minimize the entry of bacteria.

Physics and Chemistry

- ❑ Pressure is related with all needle injection. When injection is drawn from an ampule or vial into a syringe, the needle is put into the fluid and the piston is pulled back.
- ❑ Pressure in the tissue is greater than in the capillaries, so that the fluid is forced into the capillaries.
- ❑ Fluid tends to flow an area of low pressure.
- ❑ Deep injection of fluid leads to fast absorption. Intramuscular injection is absorbed faster than the subcutaneous and intradermal injections.
- ❑ Massage, stimulate circulation and improve the absorption of drugs.
- ❑ Drugs having the same osmotic pressure as the blood is absorbed more quickly than the other fluids.
- ❑ Water soluble drugs are absorbed more quickly than the oily drugs.

Pharmacology

- ❑ Various classes of drugs are given through injections such as remedial, preventive, diagnostic, palliative and so on.
- ❑ Insulin is always administered by subcutaneous because insulin is destroyed by the digestive enzymes in the stomach.
- ❑ Penicillin is usually given intramuscular because gastric juice destroys its effectiveness.
- ❑ Substitutional therapies are also given by injection such as vitamins, minerals, fluids and so on.

Psychology

- ❑ Explain the procedure to the patient to gain confidence.
- ❑ Clear all the doubts in simple language to relief fear and anxiety.
- ❑ Comfortable positioning relaxes the patient.

Points to Remember

- ❑ Explain what is the injection administer to the patient?
- ❑ What are the benefits or actions of that injection?

NOTES

CHAPTER 2

Administering an Intramuscular Injection

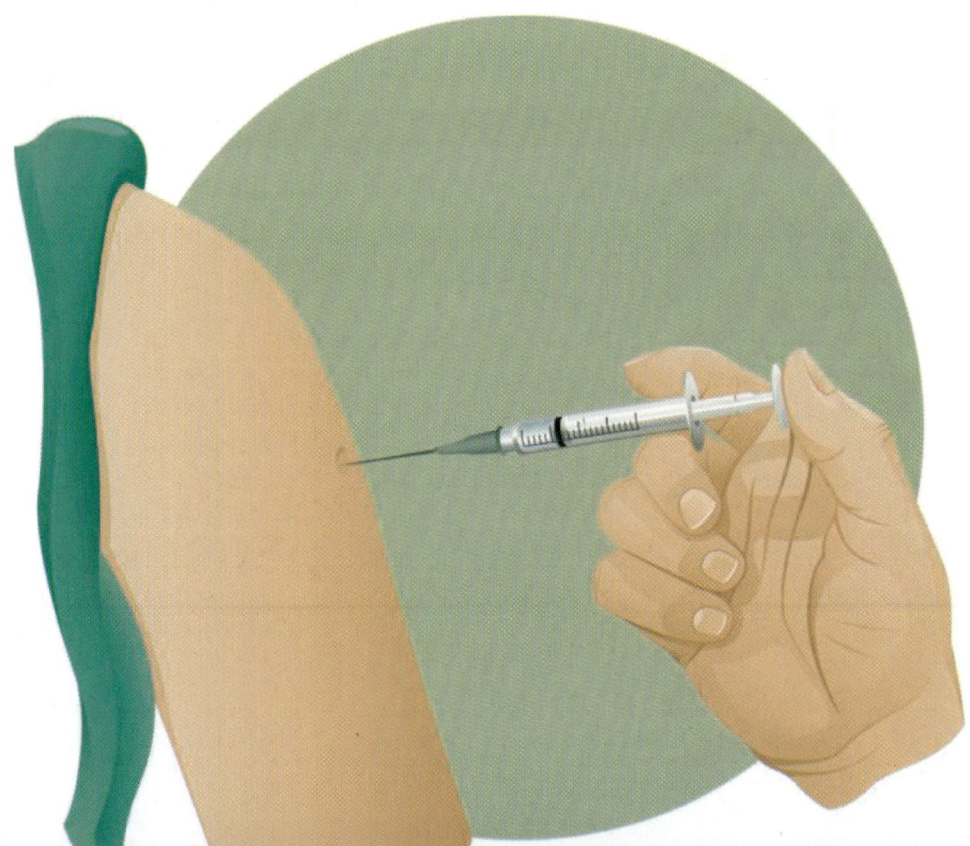

DEFINITION

Intramuscular injection is defined as the administration of medicine into deep muscle tissue.

PURPOSES

- ❑ To relieve symptoms of illness.
- ❑ To obtain quick effect of medicine.
- ❑ For prevention of diseases.
- ❑ To promote health.
- ❑ To obtain maximum effect of drug even when the patient is unconscious, unable to swallow or uncooperative.

CONTRAINDICATIONS

- ❑ Impaired coagulation mechanisms
- ❑ Occlusive peripheral vascular disease
- ❑ Edema
- ❑ Shock
- ❑ After thrombolytic therapy
- ❑ During myocardial infarction

PRELIMINARY ASSESSMENT

Preparation of the Patient

- ❑ Check the physician order for medicine
- ❑ Identify the right patient
- ❑ Explain the procedure to the patient to gain cooperation and to reduce anxiety of the patient.

Preparation of the Articles and their Purposes

Articles	Purposes
A tray containing: ❑ Sterile syringe and needles depend upon the site of insertion ❑ Pediatric—Needle strength (7/8"–11/4") needle gauge (22–25G) ❑ Adults—Needle strength (1"–11/2") needle gauge (19–25G)	❑ To inject medicine
❑ Clean gloves	❑ To prevent cross infection
❑ Kidney tray	❑ To collect wet waste
❑ Paper bag	❑ To collect solid/dry waste
❑ Prescribed medicine	
❑ Spirit swabs	❑ To clean the site of injection
❑ Bowl with dry cotton swab	❑ To apply on the site after injection
❑ Medication card	❑ To avoid medication error

STEPS OF PROCEDURE AND RATIONALE

Steps	Rationale
❏ Explain the procedure to the patient or relatives ❏ Follow the rights of medication administration including the expiry date and any change in the color and consistency of the drug	
❏ Wash hands	
❏ Prepare the medication (from vial or ampoule) ❏ Dissolve medicine as per order ❏ Calculate the prescribed dose to be administered	❏ To ensure correct administration of medicine
❏ Select the injection site and appropriate needle and syringe size	❏ An average adults deltoid muscle can absorb 0.5–1 mL and gluteal muscle can absorb 1–4 mL
❏ Three checks of medication just prior to administration (from case file, medication card and medicine). Call patient by name to reconfirm	❏ To ensure correct administration of medicine
❏ Provide privacy depending upon site chosen	❏ To promote comfort

Sites of intramuscular injection is depicted below in Figures 1A to D:

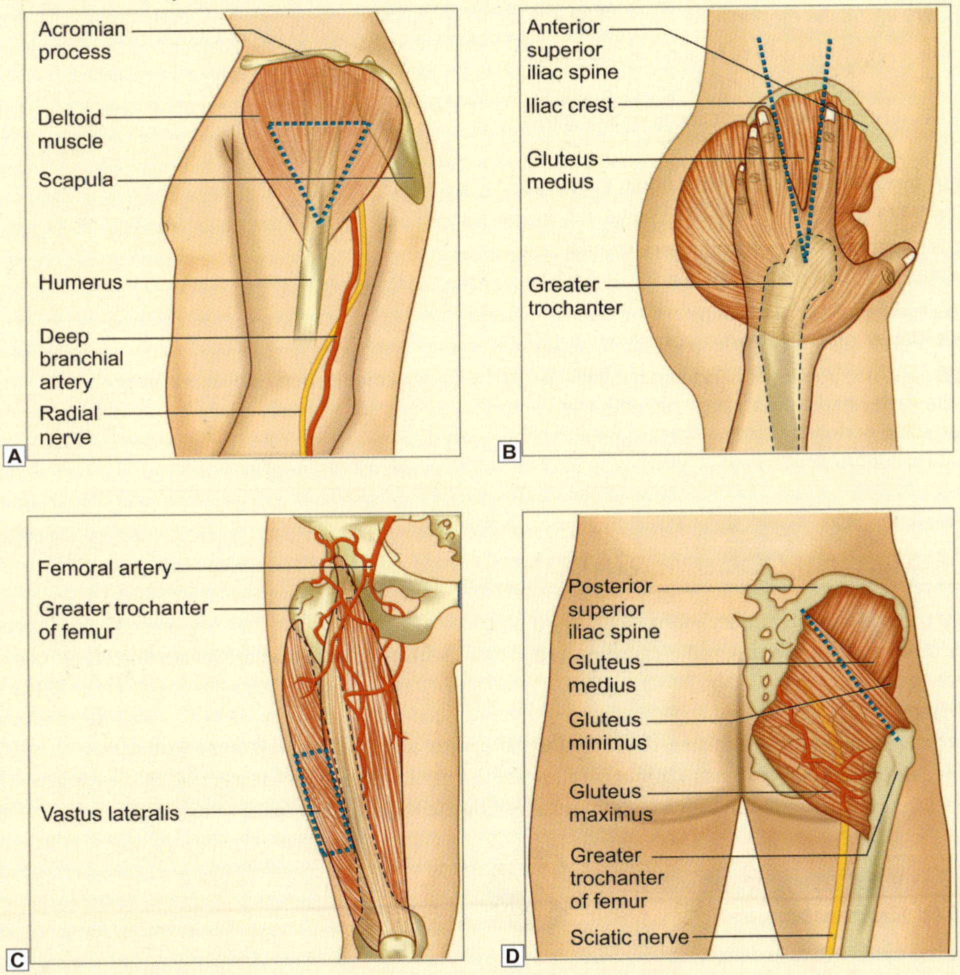

A. Acromian process, Deltoid muscle, Scapula, Humerus, Deep branchial artery, Radial nerve

B. Anterior superior iliac spine, Iliac crest, Gluteus medius, Greater trochanter

C. Femoral artery, Greater trochanter of femur, Vastus lateralis

D. Posterior superior iliac spine, Gluteus medius, Gluteus minimus, Gluteus maximus, Greater trochanter of femur, Sciatic nerve

FIGS 1A TO D: Sites of intramuscular injection. **A.** Deltoid; **B.** Ventrogluteal; **C.** Vastus lateralis and **D.** Dorsogluteal

Contd...

Administering an Intramuscular Injection

Steps	Rationale
❑ Wash hands	❑ Reduce spread of infection
❑ Don gloves	❑ Protect from risk of infection
❑ Position (supine, lateral, prone) the patient depending upon the site chosen. If ventrogluteal, give lateral position with upper leg flexed or prone with toe in position	❑ For easy access and muscle relaxation
❑ Withdraw medicine from vial by inserting the needle into vial through rubber stopper. Clean the rubber stopper with spirit swab before inserting the needle into it	❑ Spirit swabs helps to prevent contamination
❑ Expel air bubbles from the syringe by pushing and pulling the plunger of syringe.	❑ To prevent air entry into the muscles
❑ Change the needle	
❑ Hold syringe between thumb and forefinger of dominant hand with bevel of needle pointing up	❑ Provide easy access and less painful entry into the muscles.
❑ Clean the site with antiseptic swab from center to periphery in circular motion	
❑ Hold the dry cotton swab between the third and fourth fingers of the nondominant hand	
❑ Remove needle cover without contaminating the needle.	
❑ Slightly pinch the skin area surrounding the injection site	
❑ Hold the syringe like a pen and pierce the skin at a 90° angle, do not move the syringe.	
❑ Pull back the plunger and aspirate. If no blood comes, slowly inject the medication.	
❑ Remove the nondominant hand and quickly withdraw the needle. Apply pressure with dry cotton swab or do gentle massage.	❑ Allow medication to disperse evenly.
❑ Assist the patient to be comfortable.	❑ To reduce discomfort.

AFTER CARE AND DOCUMENTATION

❑ Take articles to the dirty utility room.
❑ Discard the waste materials and clean the used articles with soap and water. Replace the waste materials in proper space.
❑ Wash hands.
❑ Record the medication administered, route, dose, site, time and all in nurse's notes with sign.
❑ Observe the patient for at least 15 minutes following the injection for signs of reaction of the drug.
❑ Notice for any skin conditions such as redness, swelling, itching, tingling, pain or discomfort.

Points to Remember

❑ Allow the patient to take deep breath.
❑ Divert the mind of the patient.
❑ Gently massage at the site of injection.

CHAPTER 3

Administering an Intradermal Injection

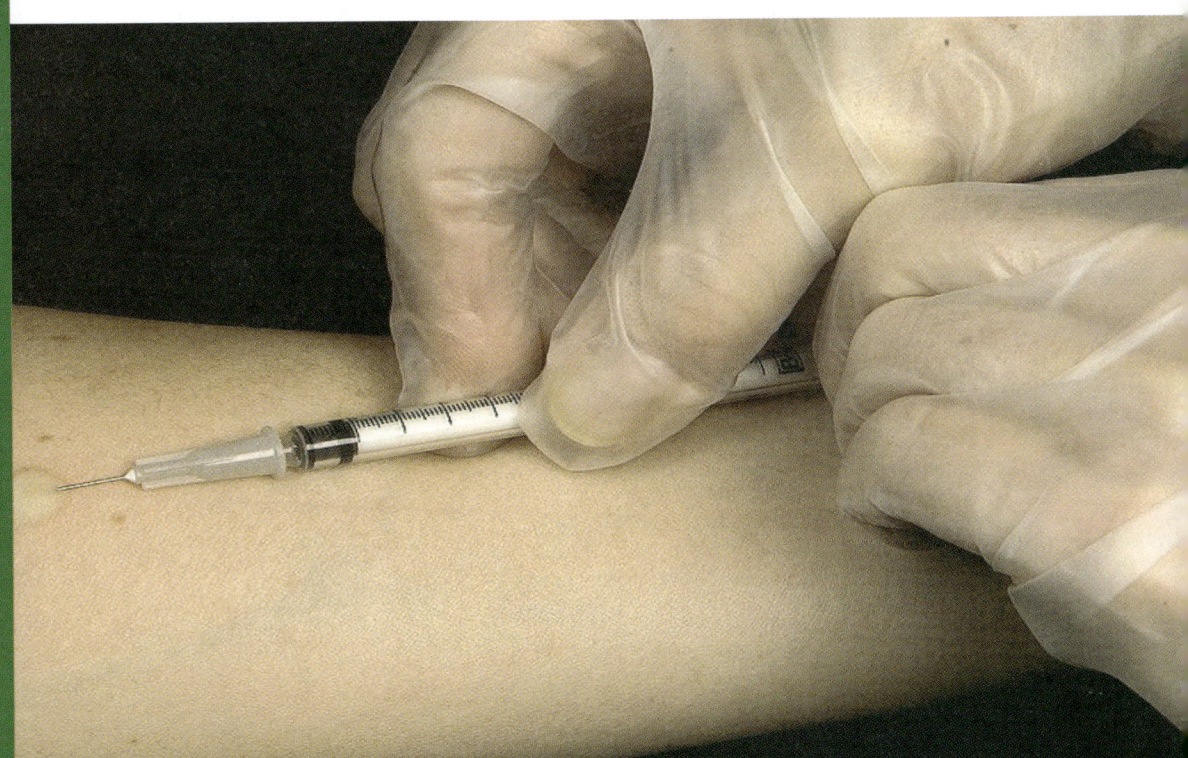

DEFINITION

It is an administration of medicine into the dermal layer of skin.

PURPOSES

❑   To perform purified protein derivative (Tuberculin) test.
❑   To do sensitivity test.
❑   To administer vaccination.

Sites of intradermal injection is depicted below in Figures 1A and B.

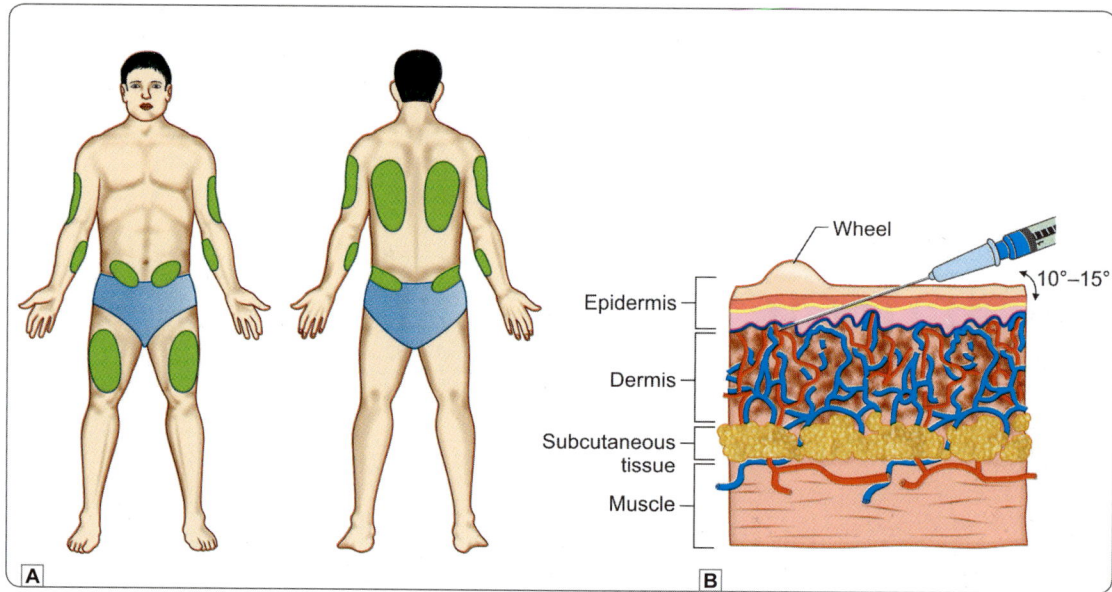

FIGS 1A AND B: A. Sites of intradermal injection; **B.** Administration of intradermal injection

PRELIMINARY ASSESSMENT

Preparation of the Patient

❑   Check the physician order for medicine.
❑   Identify the right patient.
❑   Explain the procedure to the patient to gain cooperation and to reduce anxiety of the client.

Preparation of the Articles and their Purposes

Articles	Purposes
A clean tray containing:	
❑ Sterile syringe and needles depend upon the site of insertion ❑ Pediatric—Needle strength (3/8"–3/4") needle gauge (26–28 G) ❑ Adults—Needle strength (3/8"–3/4") needle gauge (26–28 G)	❑ To inject the medicine

Contd…

Articles	Purposes
❑ Clean gloves	❑ To prevent cross infection
❑ Medicine	❑ To treat and promote health
❑ Sterile syringe and needles	❑ To administer medicine
❑ Spirit swab	❑ To clean the site
❑ Kidney tray	❑ To collect wet waste
❑ Medication card	❑ To prevent occurrence

STEPS OF PROCEDURE AND RATIONALE

Steps	Rationale
❑ Check physician's order for medication administration and identify patient	❑ Eliminate medication error
❑ Three checks of medication just prior administration (from case file, medication card and medicine). Call patient by name to reconfirm	
❑ Explain the procedure to the patient	❑ Explanation encourages cooperation and reduces anxiety
❑ Wash hands	❑ Prevent cross infection
❑ Prepare medication from ampoule/vial	
❑ Wash hand and don gloves	
❑ Give position to the patient depend upon the site for intradermal injection	❑ Forearm is the most convenient and easily located and hence the commonly used site
❑ Clean the site with spirit swab in circular motion from center to periphery. Allow skin to dry	❑ Pathogens in the skin can be introduced into tissues
❑ Remove needle cap with the nondominant hand without contaminating the needle	❑ Reduce chances of contamination of needle
❑ Use nondominant hand to spread tight the skin over injection site	❑ Spread skin ensures an easy entrance into intradermal layer of skin
❑ Place needle at 15° angle from patient's skin and insert the needle into the skin so that the point of the needle can be seen through the skin	❑ Needle position facilitates insertion into intradermal tissue

Contd…

Steps	Rationale
❑ Slowly inject the drug (0.01–0.1 mL) into the intradermal layer of skin and watch for wheal to form	❑ A bleb/wheal indicates that needle is in intradermal tissue
❑ Withdraw needle quickly in the same angle	❑ Reduce tissue damage and discomfort of patient
❑ Do not massage the area	❑ Massage will lead to the spread of medicine to subcutaneous tissue and false results may occur
❑ Recap the needle with one hand. Discard syringe and needle into appropriate containers	❑ Reduces risk of needle stick injury
❑ Provide comfortable position to the patient	❑ To promote comfort
❑ Draw a circle using black or blue pen around wheal formed ❑ Write the name of drug, date and time of administration on a piece of adhesive tape and stick near to the site	❑ For identifying exact site for any reaction of medication

AFTER CARE AND DOCUMENTATION

❑ Discard the waste in appropriate containers. Clean and dry the reusable articles in the dirty utility room.
❑ Remove gloves and wash hands.
❑ Record the medication administered, dose, site, route and patient's response on nurse's notes with sign.
❑ Check for drug reaction after given time period and record.

Points to Remember

❑ See that the bleb should appear over the skin at the site of injection.
❑ Do not massage at the site.
❑ Mark the site by encircling the area to see for any reaction or skin changes.

Principles and Procedures of NURSING FOUNDATIONS

CHAPTER **4**

Administering Subcutaneous Injections

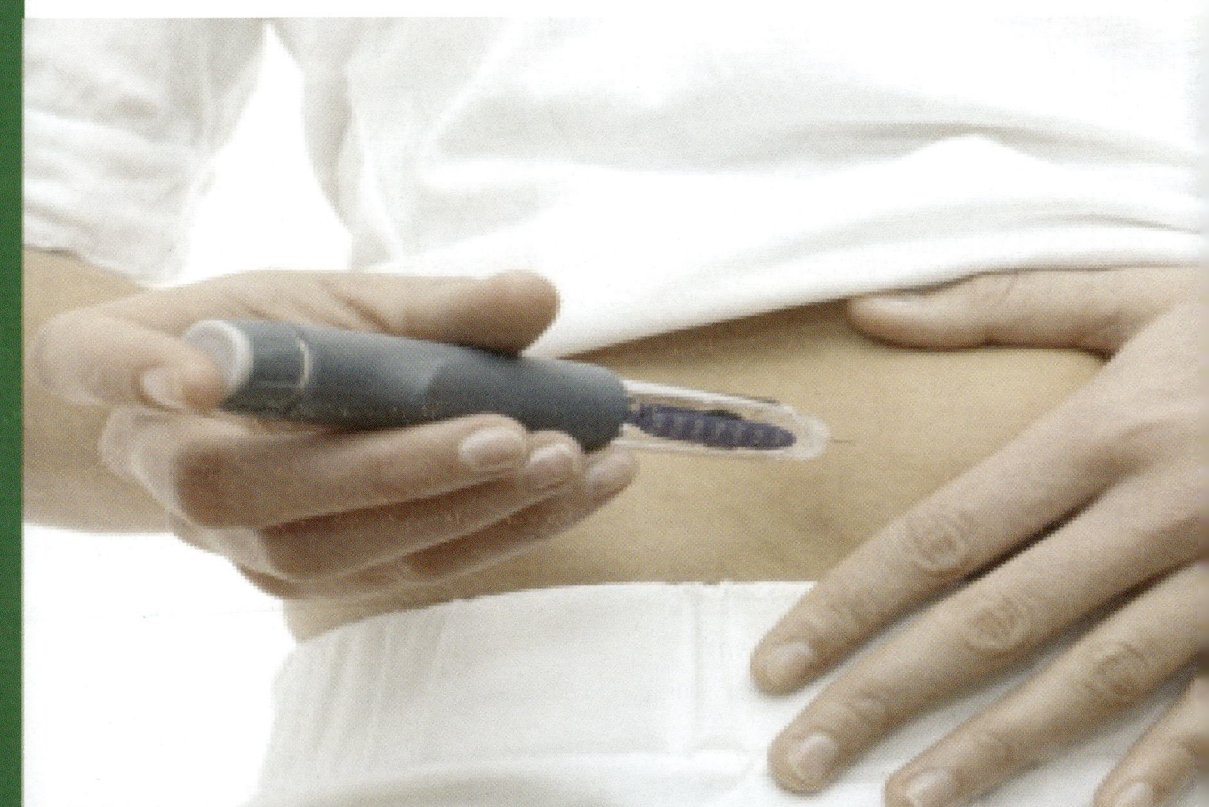

DEFINITION

It is an administration of medication into the subcutaneous tissue.

PURPOSES

❑ To have rapid systemic effect of drugs, e.g. insulin, heparin.
❑ To obtain local effect of drugs, e.g. anesthetics.
❑ To administer small amount of drugs.

INDICATIONS

❑ Patient is unable to take drug orally.
❑ Some drugs need to be absorbed subcutaneously for better effect.

CONTRAINDICATIONS

❑ Skin lesions
❑ Bony prominences
❑ Large underlying muscles or nerves.

Sites of subcutaneous injection is depicted below in Figure 1:

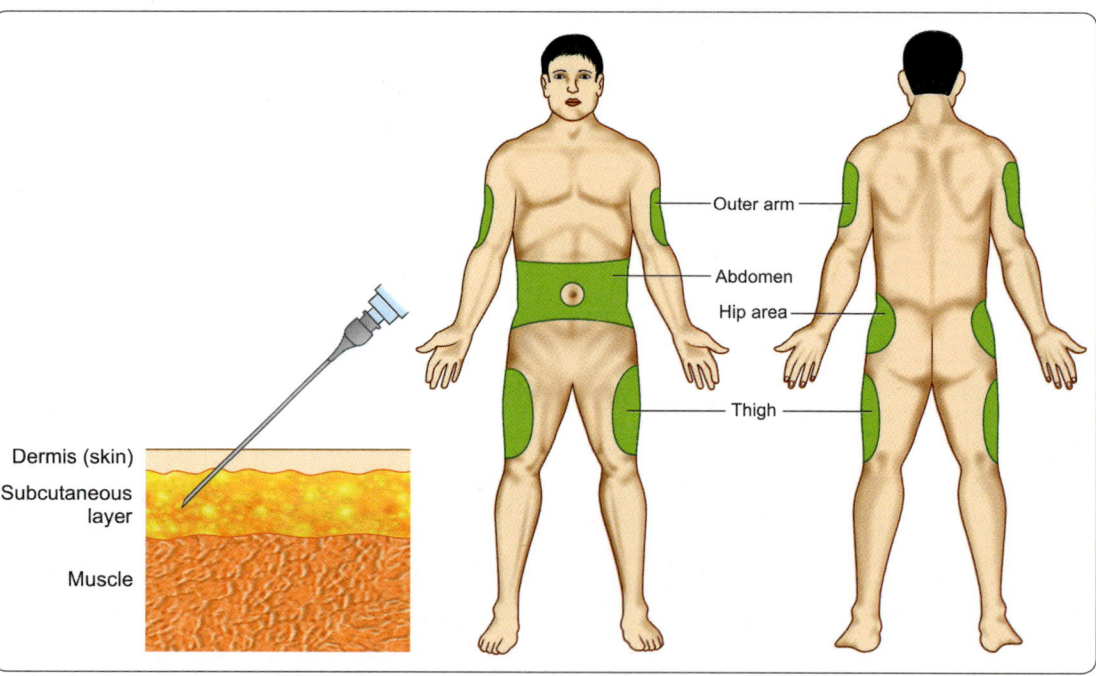

FIG. 1: Sites of subcutaneous injection

PRELIMINARY ASSESSMENT

Preparation of the Patient

❑ Check the physician order for medicine.

Principles and Procedures of NURSING FOUNDATIONS

❑ Identify the right patient.
❑ Explain the procedure to the patient to gain cooperation and to reduce anxiety of the client.

Preparation of the Articles and their Purposes

Articles	Purposes
❑ Prescribed medicine	❑ To have effect on body
❑ Medication card	❑ To ensure accuracy of drug administration
❑ Sterile syringe and needles (25–27 G)	❑ To inject medicine
❑ Spirit swabs and dry cotton balls	❑ To clean site of injection
❑ A pair of clean gloves	❑ To prevent cross infection
❑ Kidney tray	❑ To discard wet waste

STEPS OF PROCEDURE AND RATIONALE

Preparation of the Patient

Steps	Rationale
❑ Follow rights of drug administration ❑ Three checks of medication just prior administration (from case file, medication card and medicine). Call patient by name to reconfirm	❑ To ensure you have the right medication and dosage before administering ❑ To avoid medication error
❑ Pull the screen or curtain (depends upon the site of injection)	❑ To provide privacy
❑ Perform hand hygiene	❑ To reduce spread of microorganism
❑ Prepare injection or load medicine into syringe (vial/ampoule). Clean the rubber cap of vial before inserting needle to withdraw medicine from vial	
❑ Wash hands and don gloves	❑ To kill the microorganisms and prevent cross infection
❑ Clean the injection site by spirit swabs in a circular motion, while moving outward up to 5 cm diameter. Allow the site to air dry	❑ Cleaning reduces spread of microorganisms
❑ Hold the filled syringe firmly in dominant hand. Hold it like a pen, with needle pointed up	
❑ Remove the needle's cap and air from the syringe	❑ Forcing an air bubble under the skin can cause air embolism
❑ Grasp and gently pinch the skin surrounding the injection site with nondominant hand	❑ Provides easy access to subcutaneous layer
❑ Insert the needle quickly at an angle of 45°–90° depending on the amount of tissue. However, for thin people with little subcutaneous fat, an angle of 45° is preferred	❑ Subcutaneous tissues are abundant in hydrated people.
❑ After insertion of needle, release the skin. Quickly move nondominant hand to steady the lower part of syringe and hold the top of barrel with dominant hand	❑ Injection of fluid into compressed tissues causes pressure on nerve fibers and discomfort to the patient

Contd...

Administering Subcutaneous Injections

Steps	Rationale
❑ Aspirate gently by pulling plunger back, if recommended. If blood appears then withdraw needle immediately and discard ❑ Do not aspirate for heparin/insulin	❑ Serious reaction may occur if we inject a drug into blood vessel which is intended for subcutaneous administration ❑ Insulin needle is very small in size (Fig. 2) ❑ Heparin is an anticoagulant, can cause bruising while aspiration **FIG. 2:** Injecting insulin
❑ Inject medicine slowly if no blood appears	❑ Fast push of medicine leads to pressure on nerve fibers
❑ Remove the needle quickly at the same angle as it was inserted. Gently apply cotton swab over the injection site and massage ❑ Do not rub or massage the heparin or insulin injection site	❑ Massaging helps in proper distribution of medicine. ❑ Massage on heparin site causes bruising
❑ Recap the needle with one hand or do not recap as per hospital protocol	❑ Prevents spread of infection and needle stick injury
❑ Assist the patient to be comfortable	❑ Promote comfort

AFTER CARE AND DOCUMENTATION

❑ Discard the needle, syringe and used materials in appropriate container.
❑ Remove gloves and perform hand hygiene.
❑ Record the medication administered, dose, site, route and patient's response on nurse's notes with sign.

Points to Remember

❑ Follow rights of medication administration before any drug administration.
❑ Insulin is stored in the refrigerator. When a vial is in use, it should be at room temperature. Do not administer cold insulin.
❑ Some newer drugs like diabetes medication recommend using needle of 30-31G size.
❑ Patients who are on insulin should monitor their blood sugar (glucose) levels as per instruction.
❑ Do not run or massage a heparin or insulin injection site after drug administration.
❑ Rotate the site of insulin injection to prevent complication e.g. Lipodystrophy.

Principles and Procedures of NURSING FOUNDATIONS

CHAPTER 5

Intravenous Cannulation

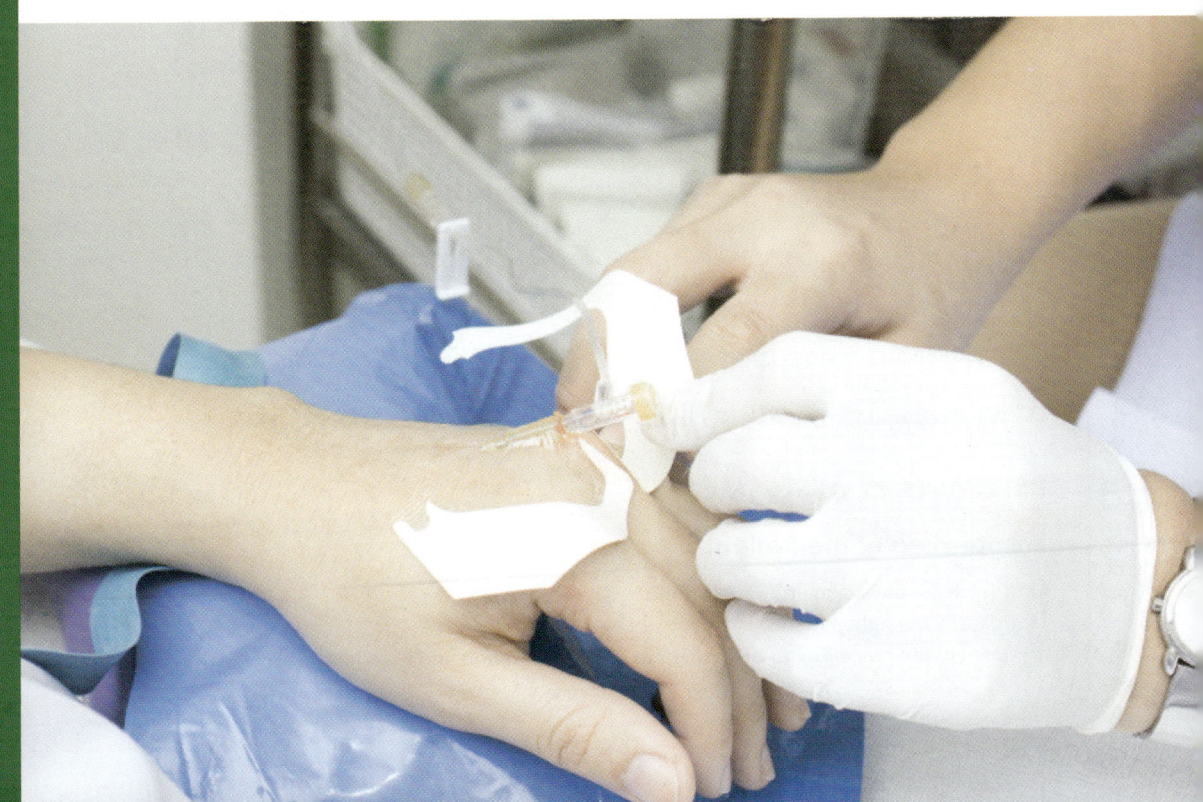

DEFINITION

Intravenous cannulation (IV) is a technique to place a cannula/catheter inside a vein to provide venous access. Allow to withdraw blood as well as administration of fluids, medications parenteral nutrition, chemotherapy, blood and blood products.

PURPOSES

Diagnostic

- ❑ To withdraw blood sample.
- ❑ To administer medication, e.g. administering contrast while undergoing Computed tomography (CT) scan or magnetic resonance imaging (MRI), etc.
- ❑ To provide blood and blood products.

Therapeutic

- ❑ To administer medicines for treatment.
- ❑ To provide fluid for fluid balance.
- ❑ To transfuse blood and blood products.
- ❑ To administer parenteral nutrition.

Intravenous cannulation is depicted below in Figure 1:

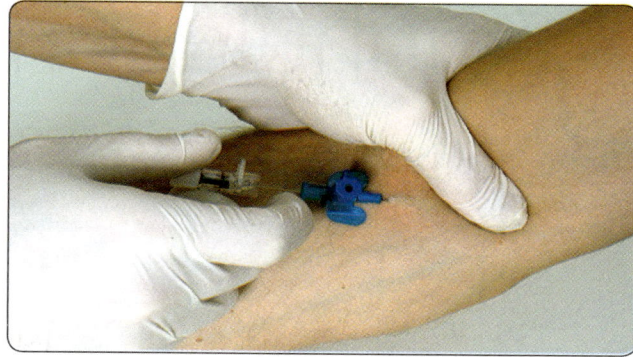

FIG. 1: IV cannulation with 20 Gauge IV catheter

INDICATIONS

IV insertion is done to the patient:
- ❑ With fluid and electrolyte disturbances
- ❑ Who are critically ill
- ❑ Who have nothing per oral (NPO) after surgery

PRELIMINARY ASSESSMENT

Preparation of the Patient

- ❑ Check the physician order for IV fluid.
- ❑ Identify the right patient.
- ❑ Explain the procedure to the patient to gain cooperation and to reduce anxiety of the client.

Preparation of the Articles and their Purposes

Articles	Purposes
A clean tray containing:	
❑ Cannula of appropriate size with two or three way connector (Fig. 2)	❑ For intravenous cannulation with multiple access

FIG. 2: Cannula with two or three way connector

Articles	Purposes
❑ Tourniquet	❑ To make veins prominent for easy insertion of cannula
❑ Clean or sterile gloves	❑ To prevent cross infection
❑ Mackintosh with draw sheet	❑ To protect bed linen from soiling
❑ Spirit swabs	❑ To clean the insertion site for killing the microbes
❑ Cannula dressing-Tegaderm or tape	❑ To prevent entry of microorganism
❑ Flush solution in a syringe	❑ To flush the intravenous line to maintain patency
❑ Kidney tray	❑ To discard wet/liquid waste

STEPS OF PROCEDURE AND RATIONALE

Preparation of the Patient

Steps	Rationale
❑ Reconfirm the right patient by calling name	❑ Proper identification ensures that procedure is done to the right client
❑ Wash hands	❑ Ensures asepsis
❑ Bring IV cannulation tray at bedside	❑ Smooth flow of procedure
❑ Select the vein for IV cannulation	❑ Choose distal veins and nondominant hands preferably ❑ Avoid areas that bend (hands and wrist) to prevent infiltration ❑ Avoid extremity with low sensation or poor blood supply
❑ Tie tourniquet 5–6 inches above the selected vein. Anchor vein by placing thumb over vein	❑ Makes the veins more prominent and visible for easy IV insertion
❑ Put on gloves	❑ Maintains asepsis
❑ Clean the insertion site with spirit swabs from center to outward	❑ Reduces transmission of microorganism

Contd...

Intravenous Cannulation

Steps	Rationale
❑ Insert the IV catheter, with bevel up, at a 20°–30° angle (Fig. 3)	❑ Prevent damage to the posterior wall of the vein

FIG. 3: Insertion of IV catheter with bevel up at 20°–30°angle

Steps	Rationale
❑ Observe for back flow of blood	❑ Pressure from tourniquet causes quick backflow of blood into the catheter
❑ As blood is seen in catheter, loose the stylet and advance the remaining catheter into the vein	❑ Ensures proper placement of catheter. If we do not loose the stylet it may causes puncture to catheter
❑ Hold thumb over the vein above the catheter tip and release tourniquet	❑ Prevents blood leakage
❑ Connect needle adapter of the IV set to the hub of the catheter	❑ Prompt connection reduces blood loss
❑ Flush the vein with normal saline or begin infusion with calculated rate	❑ Ensures patency of IV
❑ Place transparent dressing/tape over the hub of the catheter	❑ Secure catheter in place
❑ Secure tubing	❑ Prevents tubing dislodgment
❑ Label the site with date and time of insertion	❑ Indicates for next dressing change

AFTER CARE AND DOCUMENTATION

❑ Discard the needle and used materials in appropriate container.
❑ Remove gloves and perform hand hygiene.
❑ Record the date and time of IV insertion, size and gauge of catheter, client's reaction to the procedure, type of fluid infused on nurse's notes with sign.

Points to Remember

❑ For elderly clients use a 5°–15° angle for insertion because their veins are more superficial.
❑ Every 3 days the IV tubings should be changed according to hospital policies.
❑ Select distal veins so that once the vein damaged, the proximal part of the vein can still be used.

CHAPTER 6

Intravenous Infusion

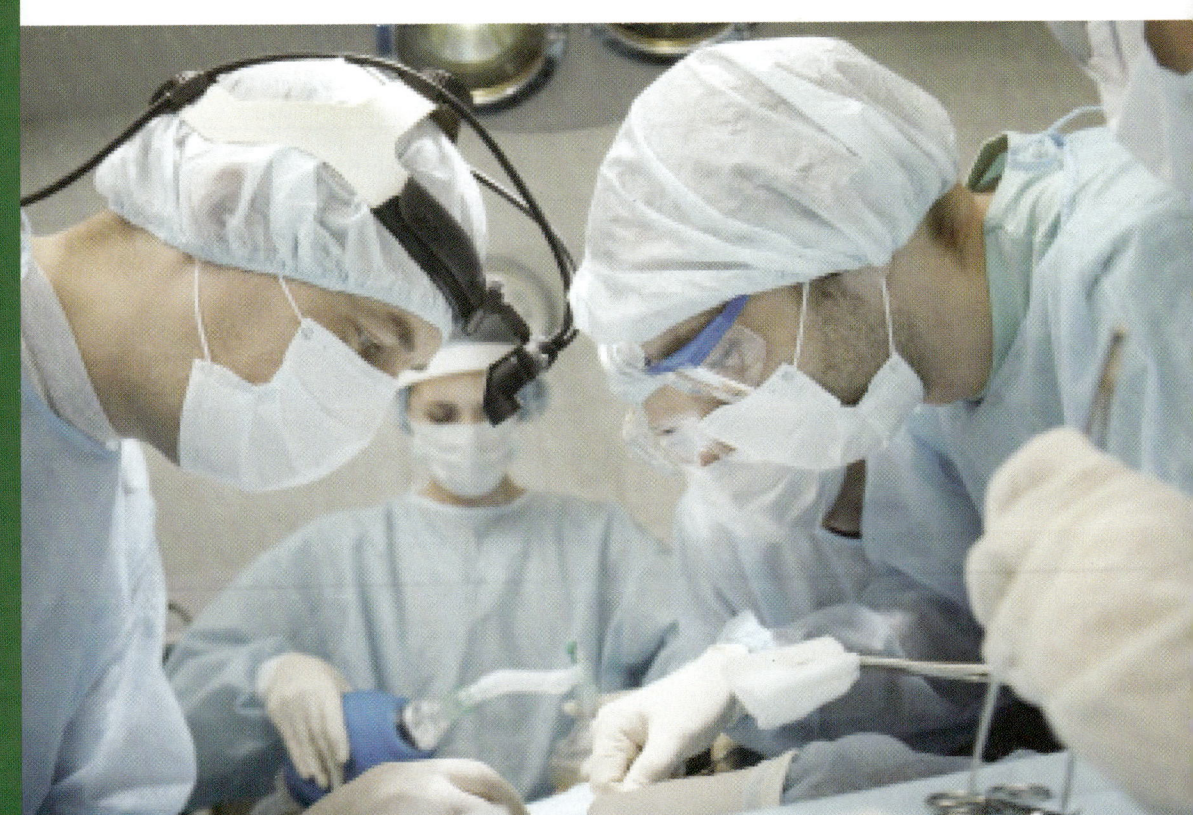

DEFINITION

Intravenous infusion is a method of administering concentrated medications (diluted or undiluted) directly into the systemic circulation.

An intravenous infusion may be given directly as a single dose into a vein or through drip into an existing IV line.

PURPOSES

- ❑ To maintain electrolyte balance
- ❑ To achieve maximum effect of medication and chemotherapeutic agents
- ❑ To provide parenteral nutrition
- ❑ To transfuse blood products

INDICATIONS

- ❑ An emergency
- ❑ Critical unstable patient
- ❑ Fluid electrolyte imbalance
- ❑ Unable to eat orally
- ❑ Blood transfusion

Administration of Fluids as per set Drop Factor

- ❑ Drop factor—The drop factor is the number of drops contained in 1 mL.
- ❑ Macrodrip tubing administers large drop—15 gtts/mL or 20 gtts/mL
- ❑ Microdrop tubing administers—60 gtts/mL

IV Infusion Drip Rate Formula

$$\frac{\text{Amount of fluid (mL)}}{\text{Total time of infusion (min)}} \times \text{Drop factor (gtts/mL)} = \text{IV infusion rate (gtts/min)}$$

Example: Calculate the IV flow rate for 1000 mL of NS to be infused in 6 hours.

The infusion set is calibrated for a drop factor of 20 gtts/mL.

$$\frac{\text{Amount of fluid (mL)}}{\text{Time (min)}} \times \text{Drop factor (gtts/mL)} = \text{IV infusion rate (gtts/min)}$$

- ❑ **Convert 6 hours to minutes**

    6 hours × 60 = 360 minutes

$$\frac{100 \text{ mL}}{360 \text{ min}} \times 20 \text{ gtts/mL} = \textbf{56 gtts/min}$$

PRELIMINARY ASSESSMENT

Preparation of the Articles and their Purposes

Articles	Purposes
❏ IV cannula	❏ To infuse drugs or fluids
❏ IV tubing set	
❏ Fluid/solution/drugs	❏ To treat cause
❏ IV stand	❏ To hang IV fluid
❏ A syringe with saline flush	❏ To maintain patency
❏ Spirit cotton swabs	❏ To clean IV cannula port
❏ Kidney tray/paper bag	❏ To discard waste

Preparation of the Patient

- ❏ Check the physician order for medicine.
- ❏ Identify the right patient.
- ❏ Follow rights of medication administration to avoid medication error.
- ❏ Explain the procedure to the patient to gain cooperation and to reduce anxiety of the client.

STEPS OF PROCEDURE AND RATIONALE

Steps	Rationale
❏ Assess condition of needle insertion site for swelling, redness and pain	❏ Drug or fluid should not be administered if there is sign of phlebitis
❏ Preparation of drug from vial calculate the drop rate by using IV fluid formula for fluid infusion	❏ To infuse in a correct rate so that there will be any complication
❏ Wash hands	❏ Ensures asepsis
❏ Put on sterile gloves	❏ To maintain sterility
❏ Remove the cap from the port. ❏ Clean the port of existing cannula with antiseptic swabs	❏ Prevent entry of microorganisms
❏ Insert the syringe filled with drug into the vein through IV port	❏ To administer injection
❏ Gently pull back the plunger of syringe to aspirate blood return	❏ To make sure that the IV cannula is in the blood vessel
❏ After confirming that the blood returns, push medicine slowly in several minutes	❏ Rapid IV drug administration can be fatal
❏ If blood return is not seen then flush the IV line with normal saline	❏ To maintain patency of IV line
❏ Observe for sudden swelling at the IV site during injection	❏ To prevent complication

Contd…

Intravenous Infusion

Steps	Rationale
❑ If IV fluid is to be given then hang the IV fluid on IV stand before wearing gloves. Connect the infusion set to the IV cannula after cleaning the existing IV port Fig. 1). ❑ Remove air from the tubings before connecting.	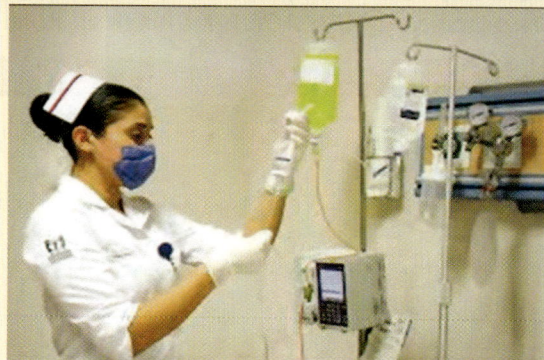 **FIG. 1:** Intravenous fluid administration
❑ Splint and immobilize the limb if necessary	
❑ Set the infusion rate drop per minute	
❑ Provide comfortable position to the patient	❑ To promote comfort

AFTER CARE AND DOCUMENTATION

❑ Take articles to the dirty utility area.
❑ Discard the waste materials in proper container and clean the reusable articles.
❑ Remove gloves and perform hand hygiene.
❑ Record the procedure in nurse's notes.

Points to Remember

❑ Check the patency of the IV cannulation before administering other fluids.
❑ A 2 ml to be given to check patency.
❑ Always put the date and time when you have started the fluid and when you have changed the IV set.

CHAPTER 7

Blood Transfusion

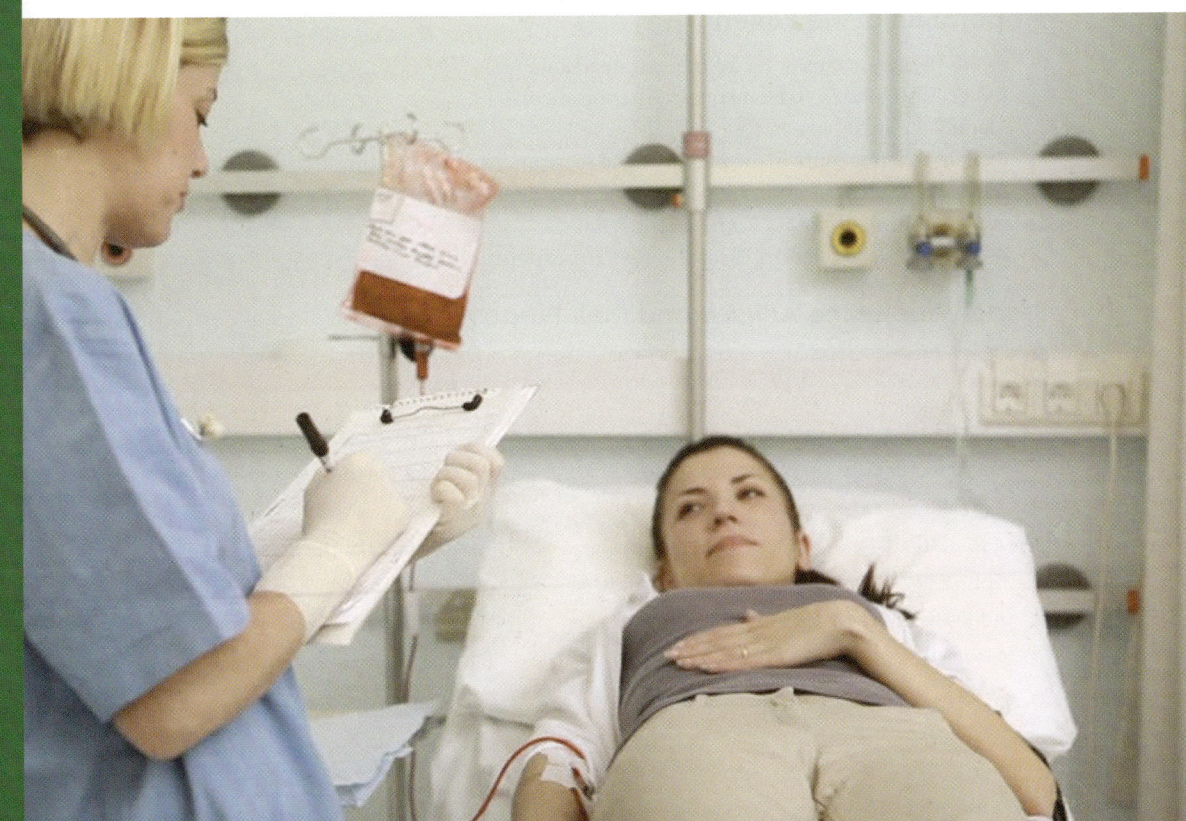

DEFINITION

Blood transfusion is the intravenous administration of the whole blood or its component such as plasma, packed red blood cells and platelet.

PURPOSES

- ❏ To treat anemia
- ❏ To provide plasma clotting factors
- ❏ To restore circulating blood volume
- ❏ To control bleeding
- ❏ To combat infection due to decrease or defective white cells or antibodies.

INDICATIONS

- ❏ Major surgical operation
- ❏ Severe anemia
- ❏ Leukemia
- ❏ Leucopenia
- ❏ Agranulocytosis
- ❏ Erythroblastosis fetalis
- ❏ Severe blood loss in accidents
- ❏ Cancer patients receiving chemotherapy
- ❏ Hereditary disorders such as hemophilia and thalassemia

PRELIMINARY ASSESSMENT

Preparation of the Patient

- ❏ Check the physicians order for blood transfusion.
- ❏ Collect the blood from blood bank as per protocol.
- ❏ Identify the right patient.
- ❏ Explain the procedure to the patient, need for transfusion, blood product, length of time, etc.
- ❏ Assess the patient for prior blood transfusion and reaction, if any.
- ❏ Obtain informed consent from patient/relatives.
- ❏ Assess vital signs (blood pressure, temperature, pulse and respiration).

Preparation of the Articles and their Purposes

Articles	Purposes
A tray containing: ❏ A blood transfusion set	❏ To transfuse blood
❏ Venipuncture set: 18/19 needles	❏ To locate the site for venipuncture
❏ A mackintosh and a towel	❏ To protect the bed
❏ A tourniquet	❏ To constrict the blood vessel
❏ Cotton swabs with antiseptic (Iodine, spirit)	❏ To clean the site
❏ Adhesive tape and scissors	❏ To secure the tubings and needle
❏ Gloves	❏ To prevent infection

Contd…

Articles	Purposes
❑ A kidney tray, a paper bag	❑ To discard the waste
❑ IV stand	❑ To hold the blood bottle
❑ Normal saline	❑ To prime the tubings before blood transfusion
❑ Blood or any of its components	❑ To transfuse

STEPS OF PROCEDURE AND RATIONALE

Steps	Rationale

❑ Identify the patient
❑ Recheck
❑ The blood product
  ○ Patient's name
  ○ Identification number
  ○ Blood group and type
  ○ Expiry date
  ○ Compatibility
  ○ Abnormal color, clots, excess air
	❑ Reconfirmation is to avoid error and prevent reaction (Fig. 1)
	
	FIG. 1: Reconfirmation of blood to prevent reaction and avoid error

❑ Warm the blood by keeping it into room temperature	❑ Cold blood can cause hypothermia, dysrhythmia
❑ If any premedication order, give before transfusion	
❑ Encourage patient to empty bowel and bladder	❑ Ensure comfort of the patient
❑ Assemble the equipment and bring to the bedside	❑ For smooth functioning
❑ Positioning the patient comfortably	
❑ Provide privacy or cover the blood pack with a small piece of cloth	
❑ Perform hand hygiene	❑ Reduces risk of infection
❑ Check vital signs and record	❑ Obtain base line data
❑ Don the gloves	
❑ Insert IV cannula (18 or 19G). If existing IV line is present, access that after checking the patency	❑ Transfuse blood or its component
❑ Attach blood transfusion set to the IV line	
❑ Start blood infusion slowly at the rate of 25–50 mL/hour for initial 15 minutes. Remain at bedside for 15–30 minutes. Monitor vitals every 15 minutes for 30 minutes. If no reaction seen than increase the infusion rate	❑ Flow rate is determined by physician's instruction and patient's condition
❑ Remove gloves and perform hand washing	❑ Prevent spread of microorganism

Contd...

Steps	Rationale
❏ Observe the patient closely for chilling, nausea, vomiting, skin rashes, tachycardia ❏ Check vital signs at least hourly till one hour transfusion ❏ Record signs and symptoms	❏ Helps to identify early transfusion reaction.
❏ Complete the transfusion, administer normal saline if ordered	❏ To promote comfort
❏ Provide comfortable position to the patient	

AFTER CARE AND DOCUMENTATION

❏ Bring used articles to the dirty utility area.
❏ Dispose all used items in respective containers.
❏ Wash hands
❏ Record the detail about patient, blood product, time, name and sign of staff.

SCIENTIFIC PRINCIPLES FOR IV INFUSION/BLOOD TRANSFUSION

Anatomy and Physiology

❏ The wall of the veins is elastic. They can dilate or contract while inserting needle into vein.
❏ Fluids and drugs are administered through vein to have a rapid effect.
❏ Veins contains sensory nerves so as needle pierce the wall of the vein, it causes pain.
❏ Superficial veins are preferably used for IV access or fluid transfusion.
❏ Infusion of large amount of solution immediately causes increase in heart rate, blood pressure, urination.
❏ The body cell utilizes the glucose given through infusion.
❏ If Rh factor is present in the blood it is called as Rh positive and Rh negative people does not have Rh factor in their blood.
❏ Blood group O is universal donor.
❏ Blood group AB is universal recipient.

Microbiology

❏ Perform hand hygiene before and after the procedure to prevent cross infection.
❏ Sterility should be maintained during IV cannulation, IV infusion or blood transfusion.
❏ Proper disposal of waste material helps in prevention of infection.
❏ Skin of the patient is disinfected by spirit swabs to destroy bacteria.

Physics and Chemistry

❏ Fluid flows by force of gravity
❏ Tourniquet is used to apply pressure on the veins for distention of veins.
❏ The height of fluid, size of needle, viscosity of fluids are the factors which influence the flow rate of an IV solution.
❏ Blood flows slower than aqueous solution because the rubber tubings offer more resistance to viscous substances.
❏ Always a large needle is used for blood transfusion.
❏ The pH of blood is approximately 7.4.
❏ The kidneys and lungs help to maintain acid-base balance.

- If pH falls below 7.0, it indicates life-threatening situation.
- The blood contains 0.9% salts of calcium, sodium, potassium and magnesium.

Pharmacology

- Blood is administered to increase the blood volume and red blood cells count.
- Normal saline, glucose, ringer lactate, etc. are balanced fluids and given by intravenous infusion.
- In case of plasma administration, there is less chance of reaction.

Psychology

- Explain the procedure to the patient to gain the confidence and cooperation.
- Divert the patient's mind at the time of needle insertion leads to less pain.
- Comfortable positioning relaxes the patient.

Points to Remember

- Blood must be stored in refrigerated unit at a controlled 4°C temperature.
- Faulty techniques in storing blood products can cause hemolysis.
- In case of any untoward reaction stop blood transfusion immediately and inform physician.

NOTES

CHAPTER 8

Assisting in Surgical Scrubbing

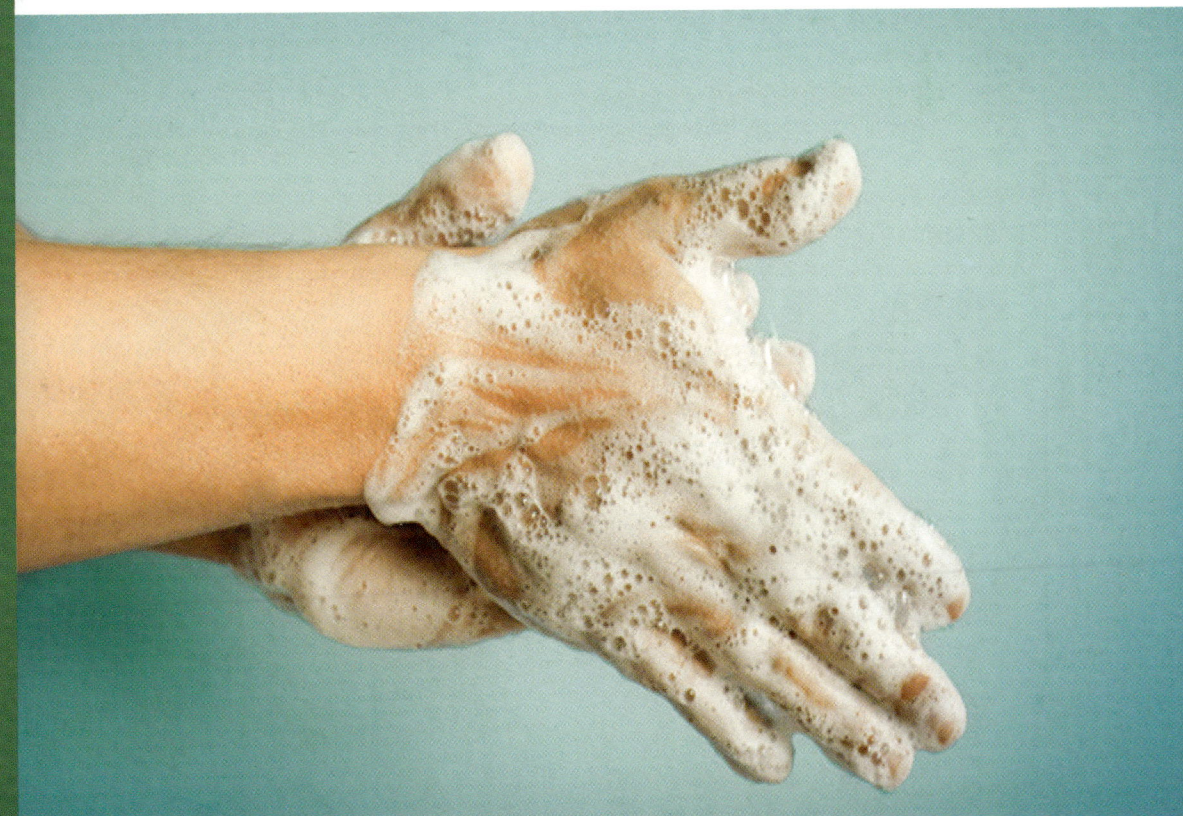

DEFINITION

Surgical hand washing is a procedure by which hands are washed to remove the dirt and microorganisms from hands and fingers by chemical action and mechanical friction.

PURPOSES

- ❑ To remove dirt and microorganisms from hands.
- ❑ To reduce the risk of transmission of microorganisms to the patient.
- ❑ To prevent the risk of cross-infection among patients.
- ❑ To avoid transmission of infectious agents to oneself.
- ❑ To decrease hospital acquired infections.

ARTICLES REQUIRED AND THEIR PURPOSES

Articles	Purposes
❑ Antimicrobial agent	❑ To remove the microorganisms from hands
❑ Running water	❑ To wash hand thoroughly
❑ Towels	❑ To dry hands
❑ Mask and cap	❑ To prevent contamination after scrubbing

STEPS OF PROCEDURE AND RATIONALE

Steps	Rationale
❑ Make sure that the nails are short. Remove artificial nails if it is there	❑ Short nails are less likely to contain organisms, less chance to get scratch the patient or puncture the gloves
❑ Remove nail polish if any	❑ Nail polish harbor organisms
❑ Inspect your hands for any abrasions, cuts or open lesions	❑ These conditions increase chances of more micro-organisms to reside on skin surfaces
❑ All type of jewellery should be removed	❑ It can accumulate microorganism
❑ After surgical hand wash, wear cap and mask	❑ To avoid further contamination of unit
❑ Turn on water tap using knee/foot/elbow (Fig. 1)	❑ To prevent hands from microorganism

FIG. 1: Turning on water tap using elbow

Contd…

Steps	Rationale
❏ Wet your hands and arms under running lukewarm water and lather with soap/detergent to 5 cm above the elbows (hands need to be raised/held above elbows at all times) use firm circular movements to wash palms, back of the hands, wrist, forearms and interdigital space for 20–25 seconds	❏ Water flows from fingertips to elbows. Fingertips are considered to be cleaner than the elbows (Figs 2A to F) 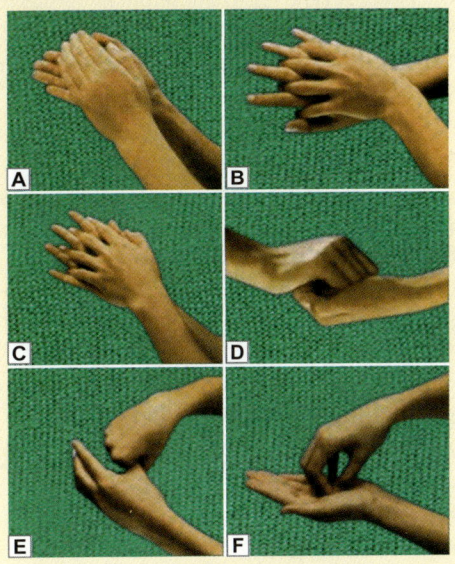 **FIGS 2A TO F:** Steps of surgical scrubbing technique
❏ Hands should be rinsed properly and wash the hands thoroughly under running water (remember to keep hands above elbows) (Fig. 3) 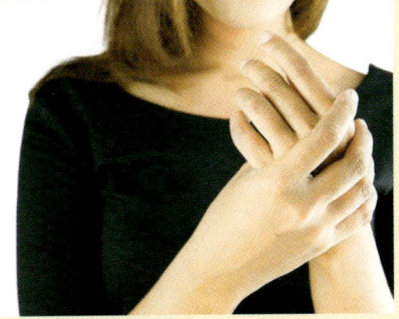 **FIG. 3:** Rinse hands properly and keep hands above elbow	❏ Rinsing removes transient bacteria from hands.
❏ Clean under nails of both hands with nail pick/nail brush	❏ To removes dirt and microorganisms
❏ Scrub nails of each hand with 15 strokes using antimicrobial agent	
❏ Holding the brush perpendicular scrub palm, each side of thumb and fingers and posterior side of hand with 10 strokes each	❏ Scrubbing loosens resident bacteria that adhere to skin surfaces
❏ Scrub from wrist to 5 cm above each elbow that is lower arm, upper forearm and antecubital fossa to marginal area above elbows	❏ Scrubbing is performed from cleaner area to less clean area (upper arm)

Contd…

Assisting in Surgical Scrubbing

Steps	Rationale
❏ Entire scrub should last for 5–10 minutes	❏ Scrubbing time is lengthened according to agency policy/degree of contamination of hands
❏ Discard brush and rinse hands from fingertips to elbows	
❏ Take care not to touch the tap or sides of the sink during the procedure	❏ Tap and sides of sink are considered to be contaminated
❏ Use a sterile towel to dry one hand moving from fingers to elbow. Dry from cleanest to least clean area	❏ Drying prevent chapping and facilitates donning of gloves
❏ Repeat drying of the other hand using a different towel. Use one side to dry one hand and reverse side for other hand, if only one towel is available	
❏ Discard towel in laundry bag	
❏ Proceed with sterile gowning	

Points to Remember

❏ Maintain sterility as long as possible.
❏ Do not touch any unsterile things after hand washing.
❏ Always keep your arms above the waist level to avoid ingestion of germs.

CHAPTER 9

Assisting in Gowning and Masking

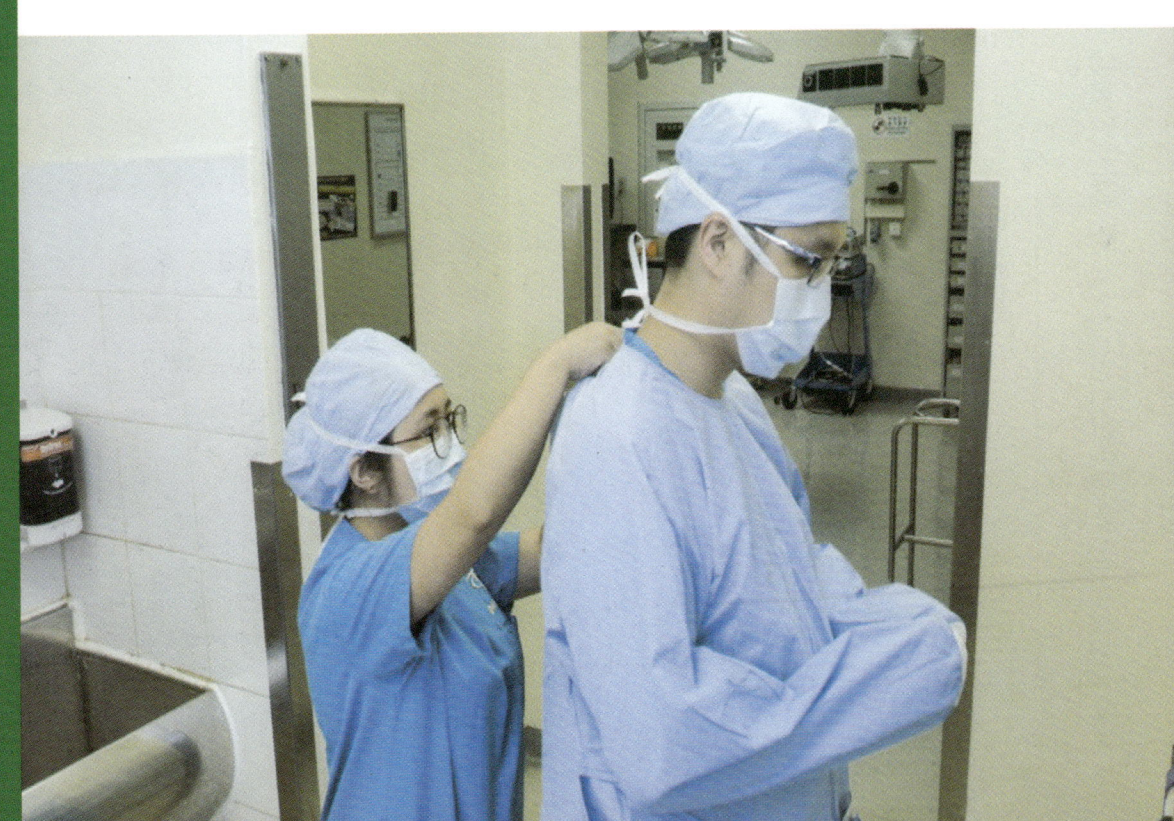

DEFINITION

Clean or disposable gown or plastic aprons are worn by surgeons during operations. Sterile gown is to be worn by the each of scrubbed surgical team members immediately before the operation which permits the members to come near or within a sterile field.

PURPOSES

❑ The sterile gown is worn to avoid contamination of the sterile supply.
❑ The gown can be reusable and also disposable.
❑ The reusable gown is economic and good cotton fabrics gown can withstand about 75–100 laundering.
❑ To enhance easy handling of sterile equipments.
❑ To protect health care personnel from coming in contact with infected material.

ARTICLES REQUIRED

❑ Articles for surgical handwashing
❑ Sterile cheatle forceps in a container of disinfectant solution
❑ Sterile drum containing sterile gowns.
❑ Disposable mask.

STEPS OF PROCEDURE

Gowning and Masking (Fig. 1)

❑ Hold strings of mask properly in both the hands and put over mouth and nose then tie the strings at the back.
❑ First we have to dry one hand and then other arm, we should start with the palm, fingers and ends at the elbow, with only one end of the towel. Dry the other hand and arm with the opposite end of the towel. Then drop the towel.
❑ Pick up the gown in such a manner that each hand touch only the inside surface at the neck.
❑ Open the gown to unfold downward in front of you.

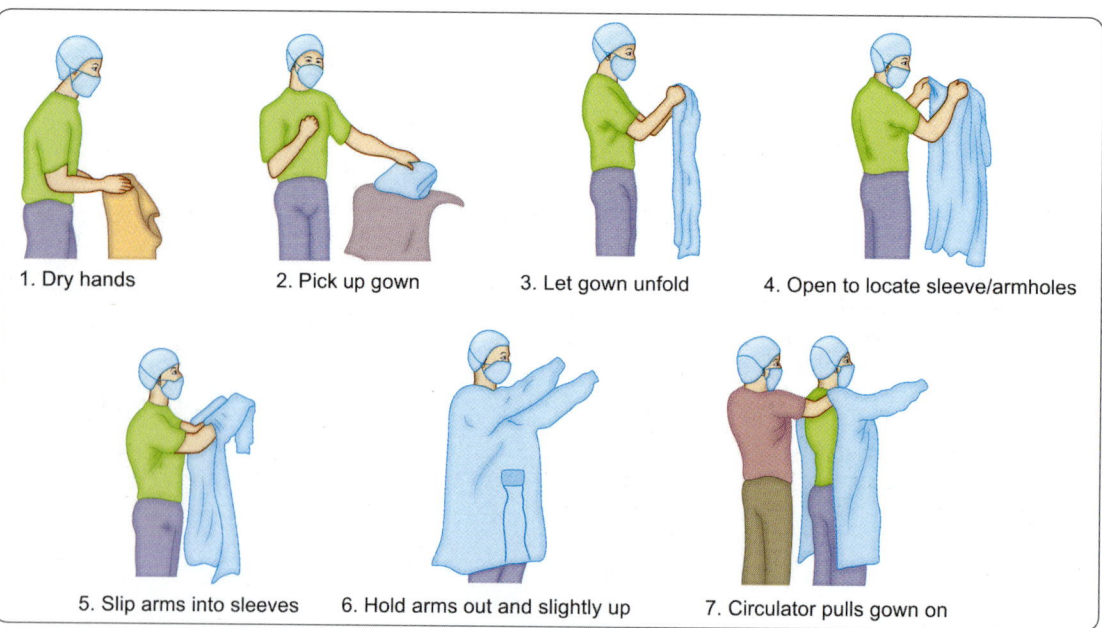

1. Dry hands   2. Pick up gown   3. Let gown unfold   4. Open to locate sleeve/armholes

5. Slip arms into sleeves   6. Hold arms out and slightly up   7. Circulator pulls gown on

FIG. 1: Steps of gowning

Principles and Procedures of NURSING FOUNDATIONS

- ❑ Find the arm holes.
- ❑ Place both hands properly in the sleeves.
- ❑ We should hold our arms out and slightly upward as you slip your arms into the sleeves.
- ❑ The circulatory nurse who is not scrubbed will pull your gown onto you as you extend your hands through the gown cuffs.

Removal of Gown and Mask

Steps of Procedure and Rationale

Steps of procedure	Rationale
❑ Untie strings at the back of the gown. Remove gown, folding inside out to cover outside of gown	❑ Prevent contact with contaminated portion of gown
❑ Dispose gown into designated receptacle	
❑ Wash hands. Untie lower strings first, then the top strings and pull mask away from face	❑ Avoid contact of the contaminated portion of mask to our body
❑ Hold mask by strings and discard into designated receptacle	

Points to Remember

- ❑ Tie the strings properly so that it should not become loose.
- ❑ Use towel clips if the strings are not proper.
- ❑ Avoid contact with the infected area of the mask or gown.

NOTES

CHAPTER 10

Gloving

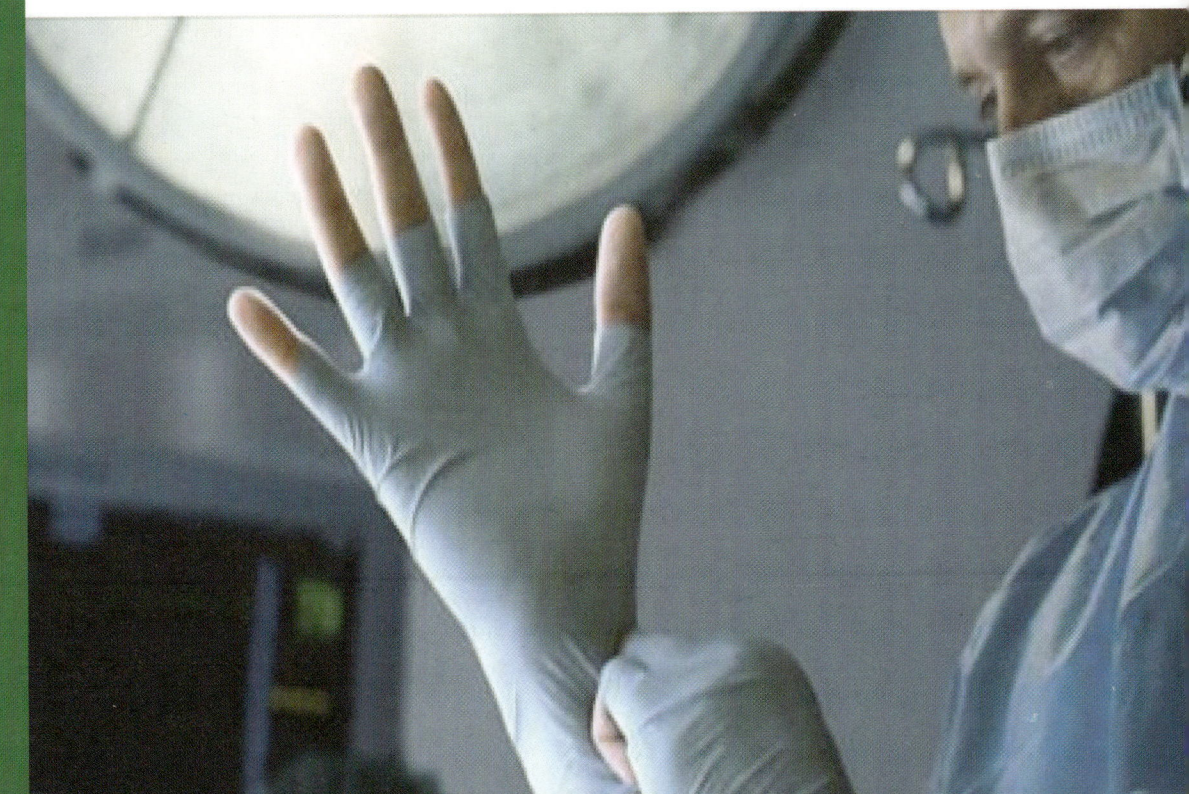

DEFINITION

Gloving is defined as the donning of a pair of sterile gloves to protect one's hands from pathogenic microorganisms and to avoid contamination of a sterile area by hand.

PURPOSES

- ☐ To protect the nurse from pathogenic microorganisms.
- ☐ To handle sterile articles without contaminating.

ARTICLES REQUIRED

- ☐ Soap/antiseptic detergent
- ☐ Running warm water
- ☐ Nail brush in antiseptic lotion
- ☐ Towel (sterile)
- ☐ Pair of sterile gloves (Fig. 1).

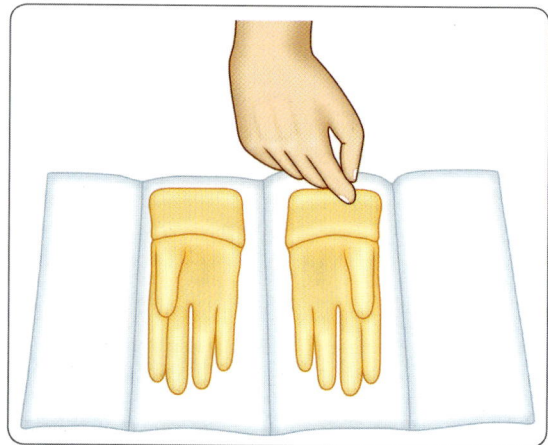

FIG. 1: Pair of sterile gloves

- ☐ Wear the right glove with your left hand and slowly push your fingers gently into the gloves until it properly gets fit over the thumb. Make sure that your left hand should only touch the folded part of the glove so that rest of the glove remains sterile (Fig. 2).

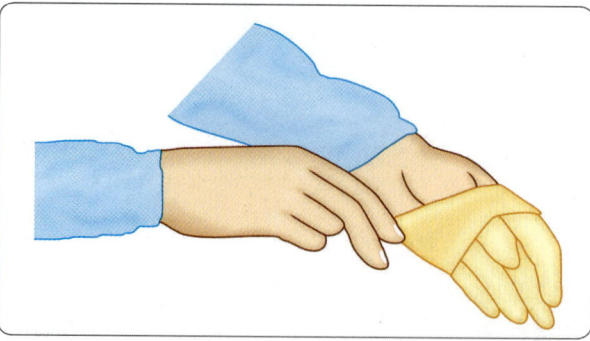

FIG. 2: Wearing the gloves

- ☐ To wear left glove slowly slide your fingertips into the folded cuff of the left glove see that other area should remain sterile (Figs 3A and B).

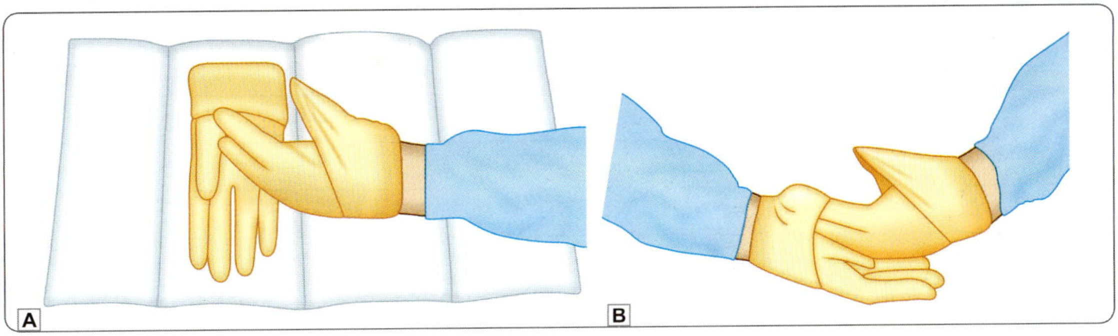

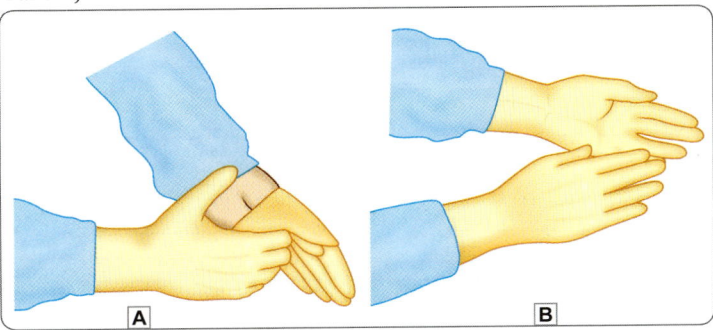

FIGS 3A AND B:

❑ After wearing both the gloves use left hand to hold the folded cuff of the right glove to cover the wrist part of the gown (Figs 4A and B).

FIGS 4A AND B:

❑ Put your fingers of the gloved right hand under the cuff of the partially gloved left hand, unfold that cuff over the gown sleeves. See that your gloved finger should not touch bare forearm or wrist.

REMOVAL OF GLOVES

Steps of Procedure and Rationale

Steps	Rationale
❑ Removal of first glove by grasping it on its palmar surface taking care to avoid touching wrist	❑ This keeps the soiled parts of the used gloves from touching the skin of the wrist/hand
❑ Pull the first glove completely off by inverting or rolling the glove inside out and discard it	❑ Outside of glove does not touch skin surface
❑ Take fingers of bare hand and tuck inside remaining glove cuff. Peel glove off, discard into designated receptacle	
❑ Wash hands	

Points to Remember

❑ Select appropriate size of the gloves.
❑ Nails should be short to avoid tear of the gloves.

Gloving

NOTES

CHAPTER 11

Surgical or Wound Dressing

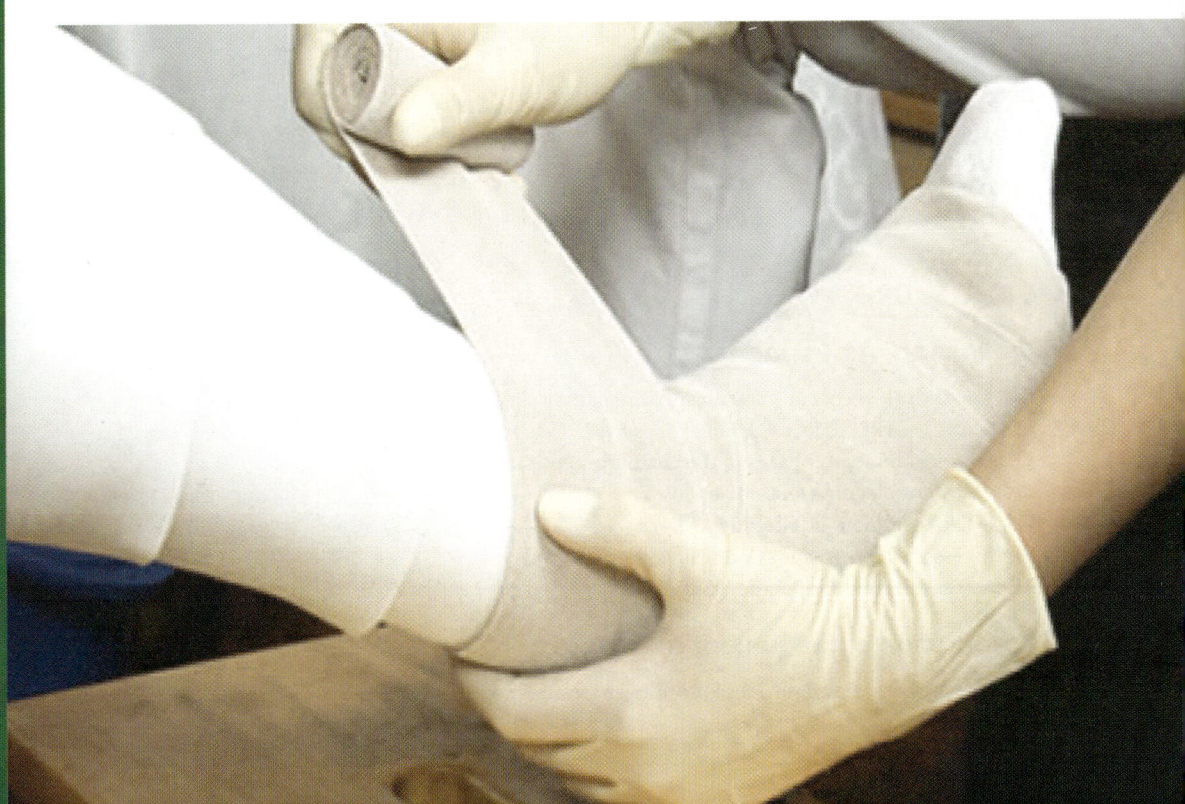

DEFINITION

Cleansing a wound or incision and applying sterile protective covering using aseptic technique.

PURPOSES

- ❑ To prevent wound healing
- ❑ To prevent unnecessary exposure of wound
- ❑ To reduce thick wound drainage (dressing material absorbs the drainage)
- ❑ To provide clean and dry environment for wound drainage
- ❑ To minimize mobility and support the wound
- ❑ To clean the wound and apply medication to the wound
- ❑ To provide comfort to the patient

MAJOR PRINCIPLES FOR WOUND DRESSING

- ❑ Standard precautions to be taken at always.
- ❑ A swab or gauze should be used to clean the wound from the area of less contamination to the area of more contamination area. Use new swab while cleaning the incision each time.
- ❑ While irrigating the wound warm solutions to be used at the room temperature to prevent or low down the tissue temperature. Make sure that the irritant to flow from the clean area to the contaminated area.

TYPES OF DRESSING

The types of dressing are as follows:
- ❑ Exudate absorbers
- ❑ Polyurethane foams
- ❑ Lubricating sprays of emollients
- ❑ Enzymatic debriders
- ❑ Nonadherent dressings
- ❑ Gauze dressings
- ❑ Transparent adhesive films
- ❑ Hydrocolloids
- ❑ Collagens
- ❑ Hydrogels

PROCEDURE

Preliminary Assessment

- ❑ Assess the level of consciousness of the patient
- ❑ Check the vital signs
- ❑ Enquire about any allergy to the cleaning solutions
- ❑ Assess for bleeding tendencies
- ❑ Doctor's order to be checked
- ❑ Assess the bleeding or any drainage from wound site
- ❑ Assess the condition of the wound

Preparation of the Patient and Ward

- ❑ Make sure that sweeping and mopping of ward is completed

- Explain procedure to the patient to gain cooperation from the patient
- Collect all the articles at patient's bedside
- Proper lighting of the ward should be provided
- Switch off fan if required
- Provide privacy to the patient by using screens
- Check the hospital protocol about using cleaning solutions
- Plastic bags should be kept near the trolley. Place within reach for disposal of soiled dressing.

ARTICLES REQUIRED

- Artery clamp
- Non-toothed thumb forceps
- Cotton balls
- Gauze pieces
- Pads
- Sterile dressing set containing:
  - Dressing cup (1)
  - K-basin

OTHER ARTICLES

- Scissors
- Sterile gloves (1 pair)
- Plastic bag for waste disposal
- Pad drum with sterile dressing pads and gauze pieces
- Towel or pad and mackintosh
- Kidney tray
- Sterile scissor (if needed)
- Cheatle forceps
- Ether
- Cleaning solution prescribed
- Sterile saline
- Prescribed solution for dressing wound
- Adhesive or nonallergic tape

STEPS OF PROCEDURE AND RATIONALE

Steps	Rationale
Identify the patient	
Inform the patient for dressing change, explain the procedure and have patient lie in bed	Encourage the patient for cooperation
Gather equipment and arrange at the bedside	To save time and energy
Wash hands	Reduce spread of microorganisms
Place waterproof pad on bed beneath area of dressing	Prevent soiling of linen
Assist the patient to comfortable position	To provide comfort
Loosen tapes on dressing	
Wear clean gloves and remove soiled dressing carefully from more clean to less clean area. Discard soiled dressing	To protect nurse from contamination

Contd...

Surgical or Wound Dressing

Steps	Rationale
❑ Assess the amount, color and odor of drainage	❑ To identify wound healing process
❑ Pull off gloves inside out and discard in appropriate receptacle	❑ Prevent spread of microorganisms
❑ Open the sterile tray. Spread the sterile towel around the wound	❑ To create a sterile field around the wound
❑ Open cleaning solution and pour into sterile gallipot over the cotton balls	❑ To prevent contamination of solution
❑ Put on gloves	❑ Prevent spread of microorganisms

❑ Pick up the soaked cotton using artery forceps
❑ For surgical wound clean from top to bottom or from center outward
❑ In contaminated wound clean from periphery to center (circular motion)
  ○ With the help of the artery clamp and thumb forceps, squeeze the cotton ball over the gauze
  ○ With the same artery clamp, remove the gauze and dispose it in the plastic bag
  ○ Discard the artery clamp
  ○ Assess the condition of the wound and observe the character and amount of drain simultaneously
  ○ Thumb forceps to be used to pick up the cotton balls
  ○ Every time using the thumb forceps pick up cotton balls and soak in cleaning solution
  ○ If drain is present clean around it in circular motion	

❑ Dry the wound using sponge in same motion	
❑ As per order medication is to be applied	
❑ Apply the sterile dressings on the wound. First apply gauze pieces and then the cotton swab. Reinforce the dressing on the dependent parts where the drainage may collect	❑ Cotton will stick on to the wound if it is directly placed when the discharge dries. Oozing of the drainage onto the bed of the patient can be prevented by reinforcing the dressing
❑ Remove the gloves and discard it into the plastic waste bag and apply adhesive tape to secure dressing	❑ Tape is easier to apply after gloves have been removed
❑ Remove the mackintosh and towel	❑ Prevent spread of infection
❑ Wash reusable articles	
❑ Wash hands	
❑ Help the patient to dress up and to take a comfortable position in the bed ❑ Change the garments if soiled with drainage	
❑ Record the procedure on the nurse's record with date and time. Record the condition of the wound, the type and amount of drainage, condition of the sutures etc. on the nurse's record. Report to the surgeon if any abnormalities found	❑ Provide accurate documentation of procedures

Points to Remember

❑ Assess the color, size and condition of the wound.
❑ Change the bed cover or garments if it is soiled with drainage.

CHAPTER 12

Assisting in Removal of Sutures

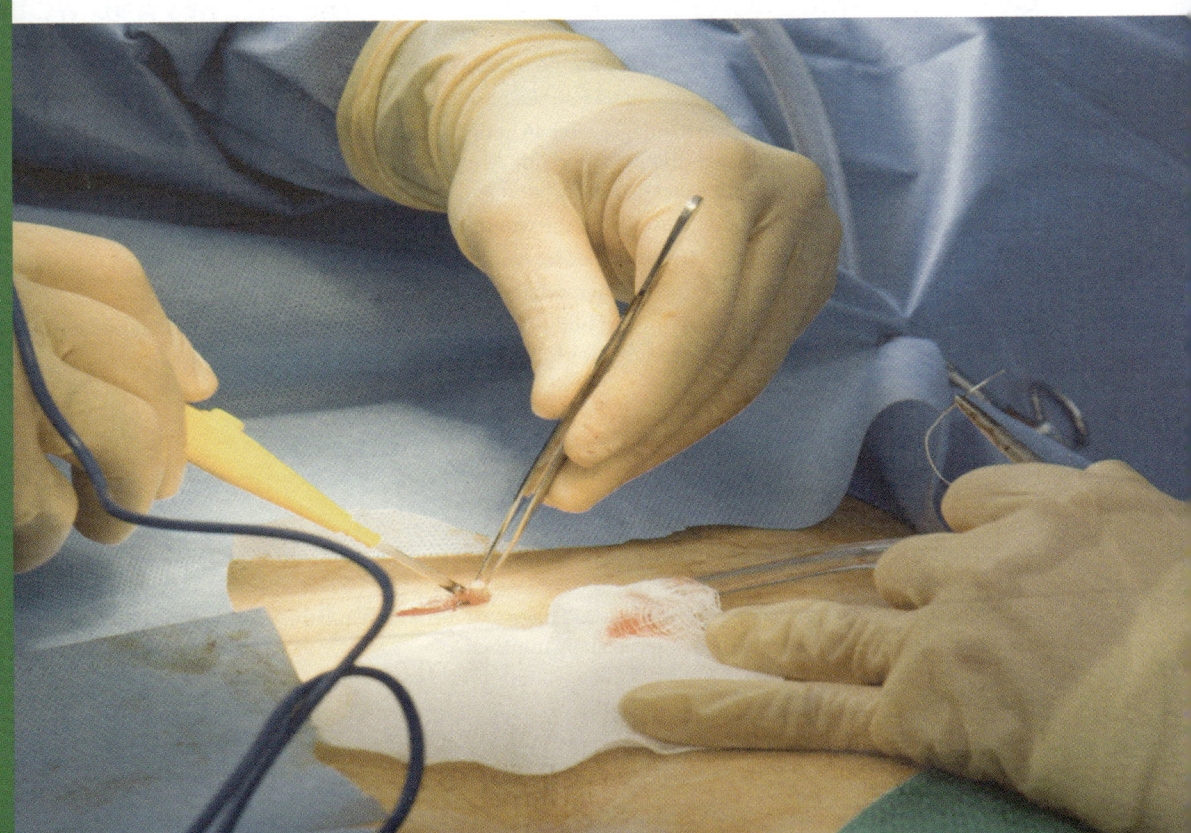

DEFINITION

Suture removal is a procedure of removing sutures used to secure wound edges from healed wound.

PURPOSES

- To recreate the original appearance of the tissue
- To prevent scarring
- To prevent infection
- To improve the cosmetic effect

ARTICLES REQUIRED

A tray containing:
- Suture removal kit (sterile)
- Sterile scissors/staple remover as indicated
- Sterile forceps
- Antiseptic swab packets
- Gauze pieces
- Sterile normal saline
- Micropore
- Clean gloves
- Disinfectant—surgical spirit and povidone iodine
- Kidney tray

GENERAL INSTRUCTIONS FOR TAKING CARE OF THE STITCHES AND WOUND

- The wound should be kept clean and dry for the next 24 hours.
- After 48 hours only allow the patient to take shower but do not soak the wound.
- Carefully and safely remove the bandages after 48 hours from the wound, unless the wound continues to bleed or has a discharge. If bandages are kept in place for a longer period of time and get wet, the wet bandage should be replaced immediately with a clean and dry bandage.
- An antibiotic ointment should be used after the wound is cleaned, e.g. Polysporin or neosporin
- Inform the doctor immediately if a suture loosens or breaks.
- Make an appointment with the doctor when scheduled to have the stitches removed
- Suture removal of different parts of the body varies in time. But times vary according to the health care professionals to perform that procedure is as follows:
  - Scalp: 7–10 days
  - Face: 3–5 days
  - Trunk: 7–10 days
  - Arms and legs: 10–14 days
  - Joints: 14 days
- Sutures can be removed at one visit, or sometimes, they may be taken out over a period of days if the wound will take some more days to heal.
- Every sutured wound that require stitches will have scar formation and this scar is just leaving the impact of the wound in that place but the scarring is usually minimal.

TYPES OF SUTURES AND STAPLES

- **Surgical staples:** This is the new method of suturing and also useful for closing many types of wounds. Staples type of suturing may have the advantage of being quicker and may cause fewer infections than stitches. Disadvantages of staples are permanent scar formation will be there if used inappropriately and imperfect stapling of the wound edges, which can lead to improper healing of the wound. Staples are mainly used on scalp lacerations and commonly used to close surgical wounds.
- **Skin closure tapes:** This type of suture is also known as adhesive strips, which have recently gained popularity. There are many advantages of skin closure tapes. The risk of wound infection is less as compared with adhesive strips than with stitches. It also takes very less time to apply skin closure tape. For most of the time there is no need for a painful injection of anesthetic when using skin closure tapes. Disadvantages of using skin closure tapes include the precision in bringing the edges of the wound is less as compare to suturing. It is not possible to use skin closure tapes in all parts of the body. For example, body areas with secretions such as the armpits, palms, or soles are difficult areas to place adhesive strips. Areas with hair also would not be suitable for taping.
- **Adhesive agents:** This method is used to close a wound in which the special material is applied to the edges of the wound which is somewhat like glue and should keep the edges of the wound together until healing occurs. This method of adhesive glue is the newest method of wound repair and is becoming a popular alternative to stitches, especially for children. The adhesive agent can be kept for about 5–7 days.

STEPS OF PROCEDURE AND RATIONALE

Steps	Rationale
- Explain the procedure to the patient and describe the sensations that will be experienced such as a pulling or slightly uncomfortable experience	- Helps in obtaining cooperation of patient
- Confirm physician/nurse practitioner (NP) orders	
- Use sterile techniques	- Prevent spread of infection
- Gather appropriate supplies	- Save time, energy and efforts
- Provide comfortable position and privacy to the patient for the procedure	- To provide comfort to the patient and to promote minimum exposure
- Hand washing should be done	- To prevent from cross infection
- A sterile field is prepared and arrange all necessary equipments in an organized manner (Fig. 1)	- This will help in easy utilization of all equipments during the procedure

FIG. 1: Preparing a sterile field

Contd…

Assisting in Removal of Sutures

Steps	Rationale
❑ The dressing should be removed and inspect the wound using nonsterile gloves	❑ Visually assess the wound for uniform closure of the wound edges, absence of drainage, redness, and swelling ❑ Assess the wound thoroughly and decide if the wound is sufficiently healed so that the sutures can be removed. If there are concerns, question the order and seek advice from the appropriate health care provider
❑ Remove clean gloves and perform hand washing (Fig. 2)	❑ This prevents the transmission of microorganisms FIG. 2: Performing hand washing
❑ Apply clean sterile gloves	❑ To prevent the transmission of microorganisms
❑ Clean incision site according to hospital policy with the help of spirit swab moving from proximal to distal end. Discard swab after wiping each surface at once only	❑ This step reduces risk of infection from micro-organisms on the wound site or surrounding skin ❑ Cleaning also helps in loosening sutures and removes any dried blood or crusted exudate from the sutures and wound bed
❑ To remove the intermittent sutures, first hold the scissors in dominant hand and then forceps in nondominant hand (Fig. 3)	❑ This allows easy suture removal FIG. 3: Removing the intermittent sutures ❑ Hold scissors in dominant hand and forceps in non-dominant hand
❑ Apply a sterile 2 x 2 gauze close to the incision site (Fig. 4).	❑ The sterile 2 x 2 gauze is kept to collect the removed suture pieces FIG. 4: Place sterile 2 x 2 gauze close by incision site to collect the removed suture pieces

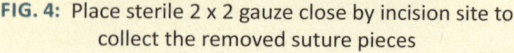

Contd…

Steps	Rationale
❑ Knot of the suture is grasped with the help of the forceps while slipping the tip of the scissors under suture near the skin. Examine the knot (Fig. 5)	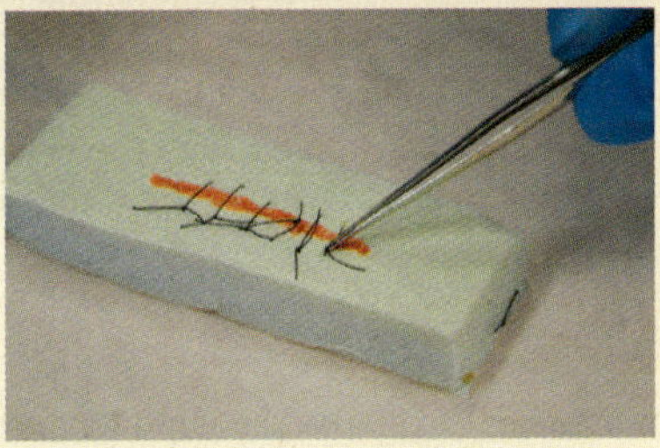 **FIG 5:** Grasp the suture with the help of the forceps ❑ The knot should have three ends
❑ The distal end of the knot is to be cut as close as possible to the skin with the help of a scissor (Fig. 6).	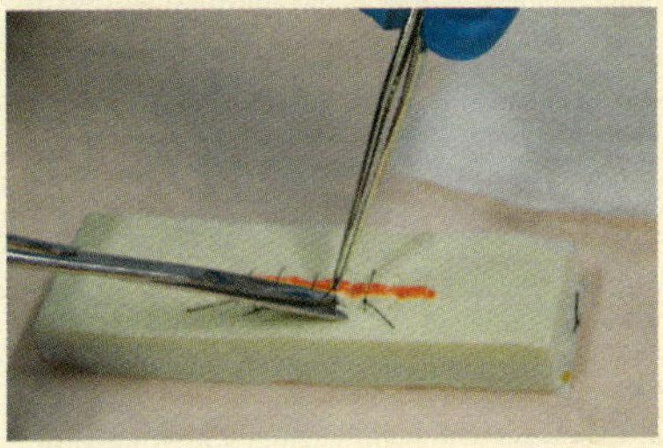 **FIG. 6:** Cut the distal end of knot near the skin ❑ Cut under the knot. It should never snip both ends of the knot as there will be no way to remove the suture from below the surface ❑ Do not pull the contaminated suture (suture on top of the skin) through tissue ❑ If using a blade to cut the suture, point the blade away from you and your patient
❑ Hold the knotted end with the forceps, and in one continuous action pull suture out of the tissue and place cut knot on sterile 2 x 2 gauze (Fig. 7)	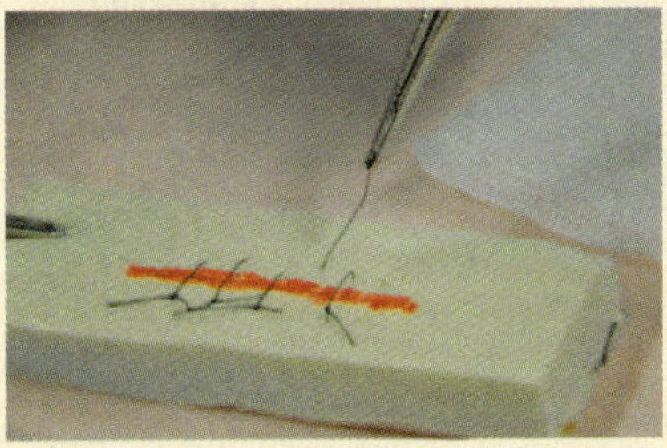 **FIG. 7:** Grasp knotted end with forceps
❑ First remove every second suture till you reach the end of the incision line	❑ Assess for wound healing after removal of each suture to determine whether each remaining suture is removed or not
❑ Apply steri-strips on the wound or clean with betadine after removing sutures as ordered by physician	❑ Steri-strips hold the incision edges together and promote support in healing of the wound
❑ Instruct the client about follow-up if wound discharge appears	
❑ Place dressing over the incision if ordered	❑ Provide protective covering
❑ Reposition the client, wash hands and replace the articles	❑ Prevent spread of infection
❑ Document the number of sutures removed, the condition of the incision, evidence of infection if noticed, and the time of the procedure	❑ Act as a communication between staff members

Assisting in Removal of Sutures

SPECIFIC INSTRUCTIONS FOR STAPLE REMOVAL

- ❏ As directed on the package, gently position the sterile staple remover under the staple to be removed.
- ❏ Firmly close the staple remover to straighten the staple ends (do not lift upward while disengaging staple ends)
- ❏ Carefully lift the clips upward with the closed staple remover to remove them from the incision line. It may be necessary to remove one end of the staple and then the other if it does not easily lift-out.

SPECIAL CONSIDERATION

- ❏ Abdominal belts or many tailed bandages may be applied on the abdomen after removal of abdominal sutures in obese patient to prevent wound dehiscence and evisceration.
- ❏ Patient should be instructed not to strain the part, e.g. not to cough or lift heavy weight in case of abdominal sutures.

AFTER CARE

- ❏ Look for the signs or symptoms of infection like pain, swelling, redness, fever, drainage of pus, etc.
- ❏ Inform the doctor if it is bleeding continuously.

DOCUMENTATION

- ❏ How many sutures have been put?
- ❏ What material is been used?
- ❏ Write the way or method of suturing?

Points to Remember

- ❏ Advise the patient to keep the area dry.
- ❏ Apply proper dressing on the stitches.

Principles and Procedures of NURSING FOUNDATIONS

CHAPTER 13

Oropharyngeal
Suctioning

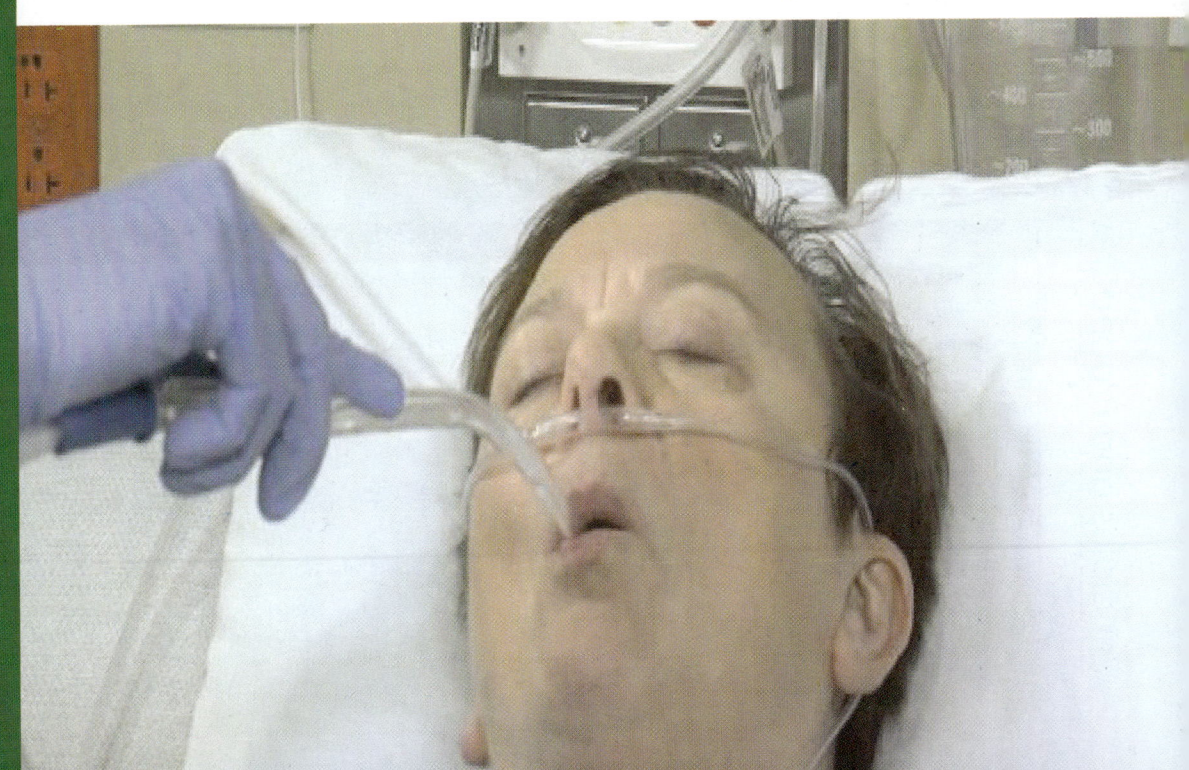

DEFINITION

Removal of secretions from oral cavity and pharynx with the help of a mechanical suction device.

PURPOSES

- To maintain a patent airway by removing secretions.
- To prevent lower respiratory tract infection from retained secretions.
- To prevent atelectasis secondary to blockage of smaller airways.
- To collect secretions for diagnostic purposes.
- To provide comfort to patient to ensure adequate gas exchange.

INDICATIONS

- Any time the patient feels or hears mucus rattling in the tube or airway
- In the morning when the patient first wakes up
- When there is an increased respiratory rate (working hard to breathe)
- Before meals
- Before going outdoors
- Before going to sleep

ARTICLES REQUIRED

- Portable suction machine
- Sterile suction catheter with cover no.12-16 Fr (adult) and no.8-10 Fr (Child)
- Sterile water or normal saline in container
- Clean gloves
- Kidney tray
- Mask
- Stethoscope
- Gauze pieces
- Towel

STEPS OF PROCEDURE AND RATIONALE

Steps	Rationale
Assess depth and rate of respiration, auscultate breath sound	Determine the need for suctioning
Clearly explain the procedure to the patient and their family carers	Thorough explanation lessens patient's anxiety and promotes cooperation
Assist the patient to a semi fowler's position if conscious. An unconscious patient should be placed in the lateral position facing you	This position helps to cough and breath more easily
Make sure all tubing connections and collection jar have a tight seal. Assemble equipment	Make sure functioning of all equipments
Wash your hands with soap and water. Dry them with a clean towel	Prevent infection
Wear mask or face shield	Suction make cause splashing of body fluid

Contd...

55

Steps	Rationale
❑ Put the towel on patient's chest	
❑ Turn on suction and adjust appropriate pressure	❑ To prevent from pneumothorax
❑ Connect one end of connecting tubing to suction machine and other to suction catheter, fill sterile bowl with sterile water	❑ Prepare suction apparatus
❑ Suction small amount of water from bowl	❑ To ensure functioning of apparatus and to lubricate catheter
❑ Remove oxygen mask if present	
❑ Insert catheter into mouth along gum line to pharynx. Move catheter in oral cavity until secretions are cleared.	
❑ Encourage client to cough during suctioning	
❑ Replace oxygen mask	
❑ Rinse catheter in bowl of water until connecting tubing is cleared	
❑ Turn off suction	
❑ Reassess client's respiratory status	❑ Assure the clearance of respiratory passage
❑ Remove towel, place in laundry bag	
❑ Remove gloves	
❑ Replace the articles	
❑ Wash hands	❑ Prevent transmission of microorganisms
❑ Position the patient comfortably. Auscultate over lung area	❑ To make sure the clearance of respiratory passage
❑ Record the time of suctioning and the amount and color of secretions	❑ Provide accurate documentation and provide for comprehensive care

Points to Remember

- ❑ Do not keep the suction catheter more than 10 seconds in the oropharynx.
- ❑ Auscultate the chest after suctioning once more.
- ❑ Examine the secretions collected in the suction machine.

Oropharyngeal Suctioning

CHAPTER 14

Tracheostomy Care and Suctioning

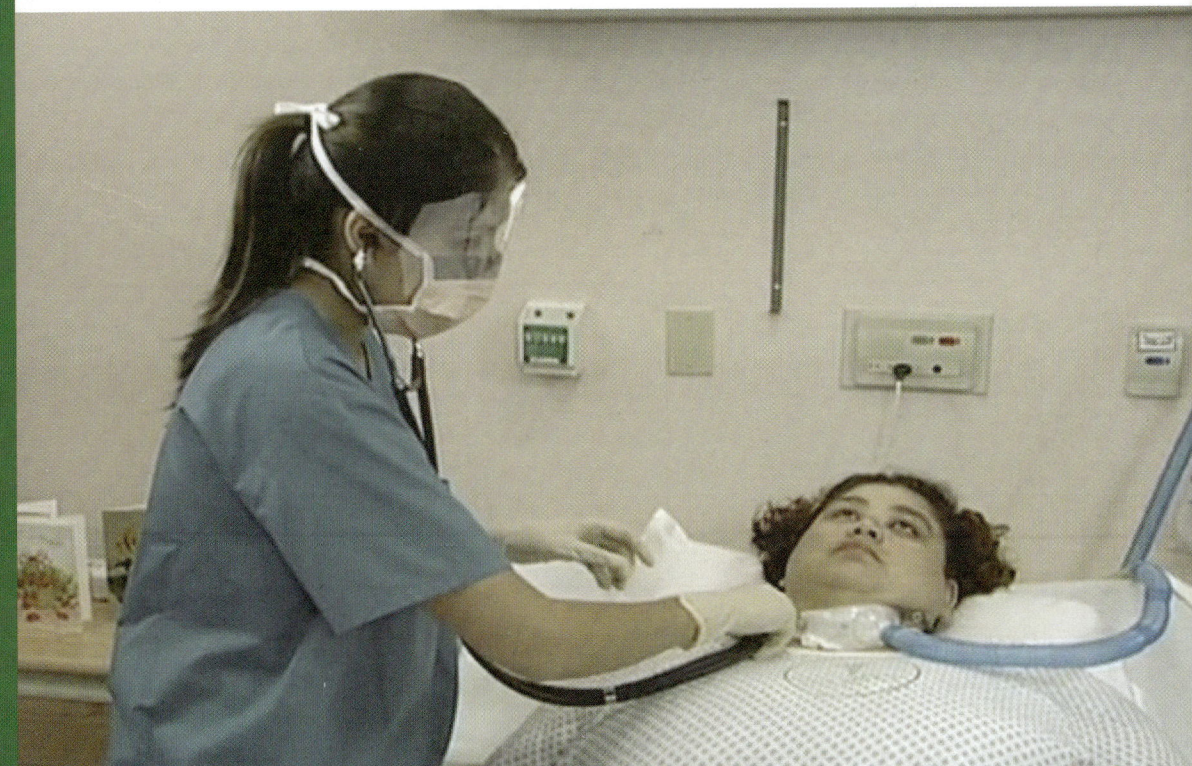

DEFINITION

A tracheostomy is the opening made into the trachea to maintain a patent airway when there is obstruction in the trachea

INDICATIONS

- ❑ Obstruction of the trachea
- ❑ Breathing difficulty caused by edema, injury or pulmonary conditions
- ❑ Tracheal or laryngeal surgery
- ❑ To prevent from secretions or food obstruction because of swallowing problems
- ❑ Airway protection after head and neck surgery
- ❑ Long-term need for ventilator support

PURPOSES

- ❑ To maintain the patent airway
- ❑ To facilitate healing and prevent skin excoriation around the site of tracheostomy
- ❑ To promote comfort and well-being of the patient
- ❑ To prevent infection at the tracheostomy site
- ❑ To assess the condition of ostomy

ARTICLES REQUIRED AND THEIR PURPOSES

Clean Tray

Articles	Purposes
❑ Sterile suction catheter with cover and suction apparatus	❑ To perform suctioning
❑ Sterile water/Normal saline	❑ To dip the suction catheter
❑ Hydrogen peroxide	❑ To loosen the secretions from inner cannula
❑ Sterile gloves (2 pairs)	❑ To prevent cross infection
❑ Clean scissors	❑ To cut guaze pieces and tie
❑ Face mask and eye shield	❑ For protection
❑ Kidney tray	❑ To collect wet waste
❑ Antiseptic ointment	❑ To apply on stoma

Sterile Tray

Articles	Purposes
❑ Sterile towel	❑ To prevent spillage
❑ Sterile nylon brush	❑ To clean inner cannula
❑ Sterile guaze square	❑ To clean stoma
❑ Tracheostomy tie tapes	❑ To tie flanges
❑ Sterile bowl	❑ To keep solution

STEPS OF PROCEDURE AND RATIONALE

Steps	Rationale
❑ Assess condition of stoma for redness, swelling, secretions or bleeding	❑ To know the general condition of the stoma
❑ Examine the neck for subcutaneous emphysema evidenced by crepitus around the ostomy site.	❑ To know early signs of infection
❑ Explain the procedure to the patient and teach means of communication such as eye blinking or raising finger to indicate pain.	❑ To gain confidence and cooperation from the patient
❑ Assist patient to a fowlers position and place mackintosh and draw sheet on chest	❑ To ease in performing the procedure
❑ Wash hands thoroughly	❑ As per the hospital guidelines
❑ Assemble equipments (a) Open sterile tracheostomy kit, (b) take hydrogen peroxide and normal saline in a separate bowls (c) suction kit or tracheostomy care kit.	❑ To ease in performing the procedure
❑ Put on sterile gloves place the sterile towel on patient's chest.	❑ To avoid soiling of the patients garments and bed
❑ Suction the full length of the tracheostomy tube and pharynx thoroughly	❑ To remove the secretions
❑ Rins the suction catheter and discard it	❑ To remove the secretions
❑ Unlock the inner cannula and remove it gently pulling it out towards you in line with its curvature	❑ To clean the inner cannula
❑ Remove the soiled tracheostomy dressing, discard the dressing and gloves	❑ To prevent further infection, to change the dressing
❑ Wear a second pair of gloves	❑ To prevent cross infection
❑ Clean the flange of the tube using sterile applicator or gauze moistened with hydrogen peroxide and then with normal saline. Use each applicator once only	❑ To remove the secretions or mucous from the tracheostomy tube
❑ Clean the stoma area with gauze (a) hydrogen peroxide mixed with normal saline should be used (b) Thoroughly cleans area using gauze with sterile normal saline	❑ To prevent further infection, to clean the stoma
❑ Dry the stoma with dry sterile gauze (a) A thin layer of antibiotic ointment may be applied to the stoma with a cotton swab	❑ To prevent from infections.
❑ Cleaning the inner cannula (a) Remove the inner cannula from the soaking solution (b) clean the lumen and entire cannula using the brush (c) Rinse the cannula using normal saline (d) Gently tap the cannula against the inside of the sterile saline container after rinsing	❑ To clean the inner cannula properly
❑ Replace the inner cannula and secure it in place (a) Insert the inner cannula by grasping the outer flange and pushing in the direction of its curvature. (b) Lock the cannula in place by turning the lock	❑ To replace the inner cannula for further use and proper functioning
❑ Apply sterile dressing a) open and refold a 4 × 4 gauze dressing in to 'v' shape and place under the flange of the tracheostomy tube.	❑ To prevent irritation to the skin.
❑ Change the tracheostomy ties (a) Leave the soiled tape in place until the new one is applied (b) cut a piece of tape that is twice the neck circumference plus 10 cm (c) Remove old tapes carefully	❑ To avoid displacement of the tube and to assure the tube to be in proper place.
❑ Document all relevant information in the chart (a) Suctioning done (b) Tracheostomy care carried out (c) Dressing changed (d) Observations	❑ To know the when the care is been provided.

Tracheostomy Care and Suctioning

NOTES

CHAPTER 15

Monitoring Central Venous Pressure

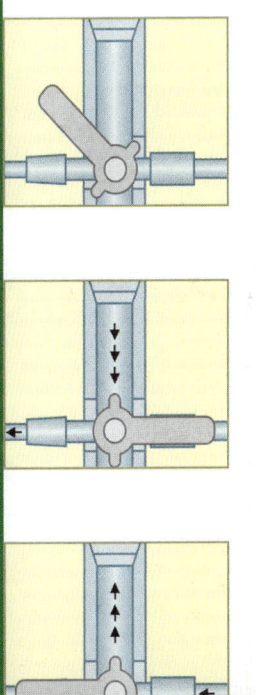

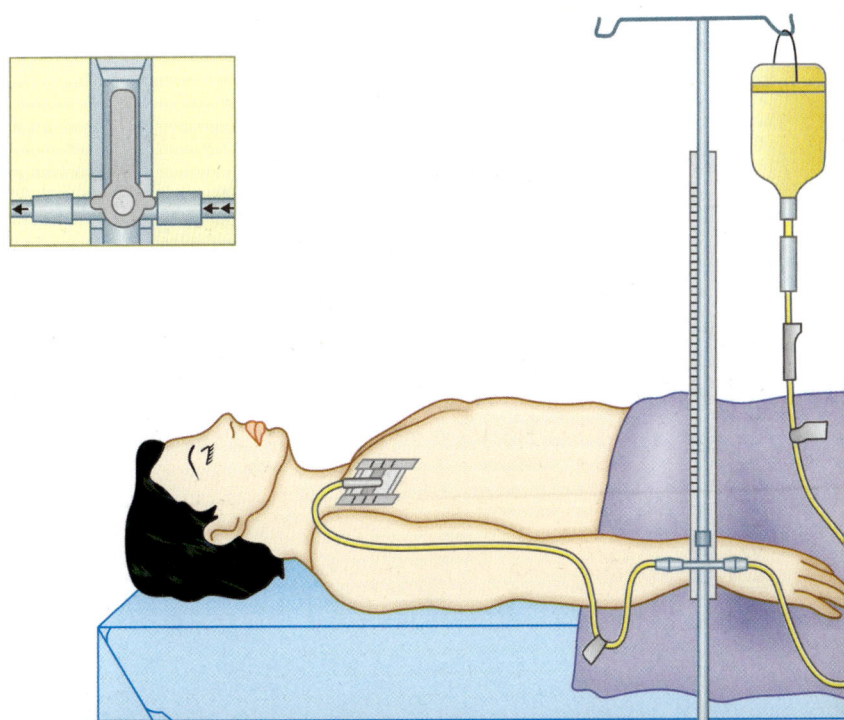

DEFINITION

Central venous pressure (CVP) is a measure of the pressure within the right atrium of the heart (Fig. 1).

PURPOSES

- ❑ To serve guide for fluid replacement.
- ❑ To monitor pressures in the right atrium and central veins.
- ❑ To evaluate right sided heart hemodynamic.
- ❑ To evaluate patient's response to fluid resuscitation.

ARTICLES REQUIRED AND THEIR PURPOSES

Articles	Purposes
❑ IV tubing	❑ To connect the CVP line
❑ Manometer set	❑ To check the reading
❑ Normal saline	❑ To fill the manometer.
❑ Adhesive tape	❑ To tie the tubings
❑ Sterile gloves	❑ To prevent cross infection
❑ Stopcock	❑ To set the time

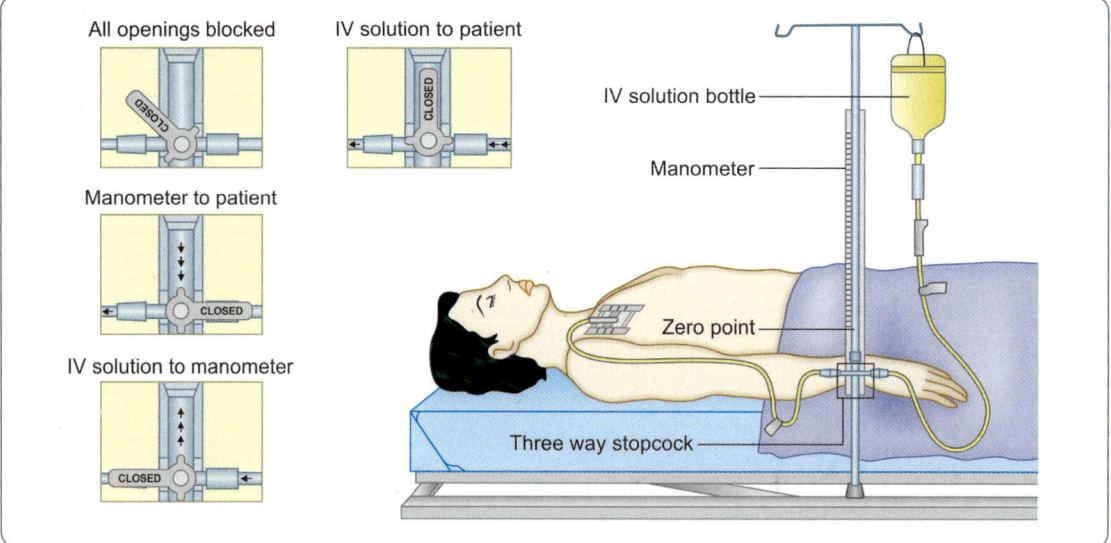

All openings blocked

IV solution to patient

Manometer to patient

IV solution to manometer

IV solution bottle

Manometer

Zero point

Three way stopcock

FIG. 1: CVP manometer to measure the pressure within the right atrium of the heart

STEPS OF PROCEDURE AND RATIONALE

Steps	Rationale
❏ Explain the procedure to the patient	❏ To allay anxiety and fear of the patient
❏ Wash hands and apply gloves	❏ To reduce transmission of microorganisms
❏ Locate the phlebostatic level. By providing supine position to the patient with no pillow under head. Mark the level of right atrium (at the mid-axillary line about 1/3rd of the distance from anterior to posterior chest wall) in the 4th intercostal space	❏ To identify the level of the atrium
❏ Fix the water manometer on an IV pole. Place the zero level of the manometer at the level of phlebostatic axis	❏ To get accurate reading
❏ Connect the CVP manometer to the upper port of the stopcock	
❏ Connect the CVP tubing from the client to the second side port of the stopcock	❏ Establishes IV line from normal saline to CVP catheter
❏ Turn stopcock off to client and fill manometer with normal saline to the 20 cm mark above the anticipated reading	❏ Normal CVP varies from 8 cm to 12 cm of water
❏ Hold manometer at the phlebostatic level and turn the stopcock off to the normal saline	❏ System is open from the manometer to the client
❏ Watch the fluid falls in manometer. Take CVP reading when fluid stabilized	❏ To know the pressure in right atrium or central veins
❏ Turn stopcock off to the manometer	❏ Re-establish fluid flow from the IV to the client
❏ Reposition the patient	
❏ Wash hands	❏ Prevent spread of microorgansims
❏ Record procedure and reading in nurse's record	❏ Provide continuity of care

Monitoring Central Venous Pressure

NOTES

Assisting in Insertion of Central Venous Catheter

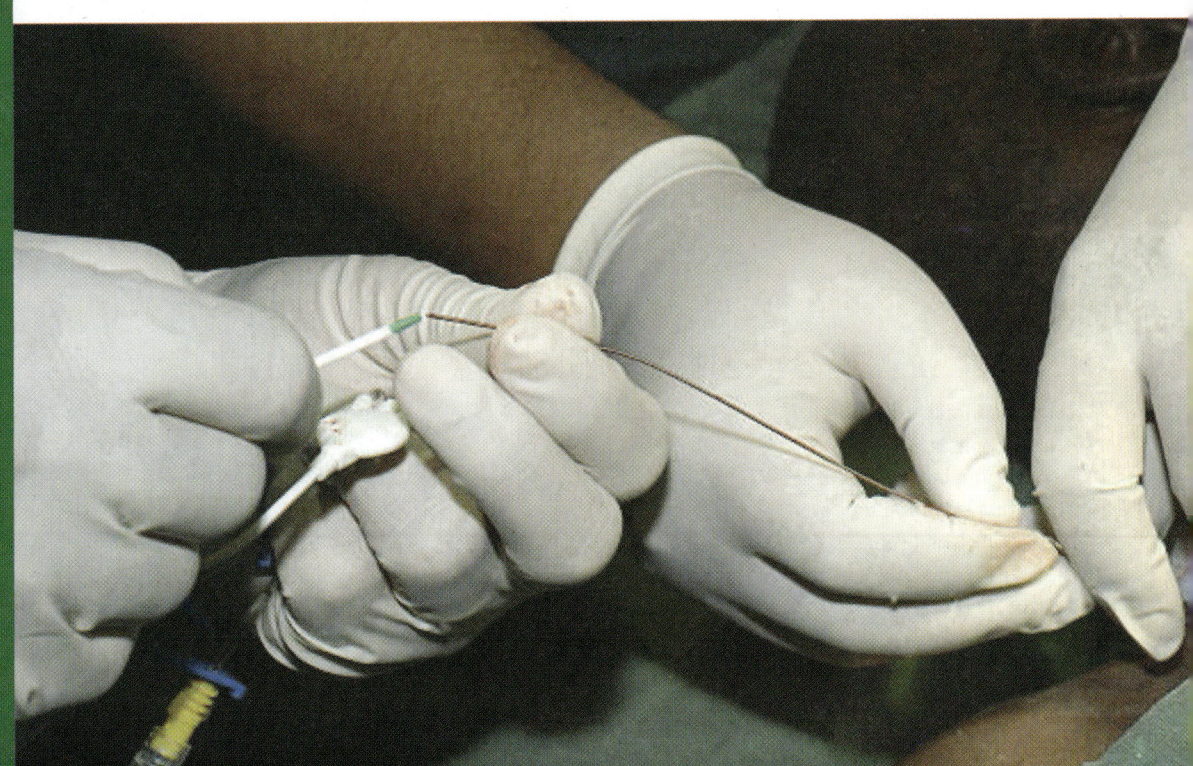

DEFINITION

Insertion of central venous catheter (CVC) into a large central vein of the body usually above the right side of the heart.

Central venous catheter

❑ Single lumen catheter (Fig. 1)

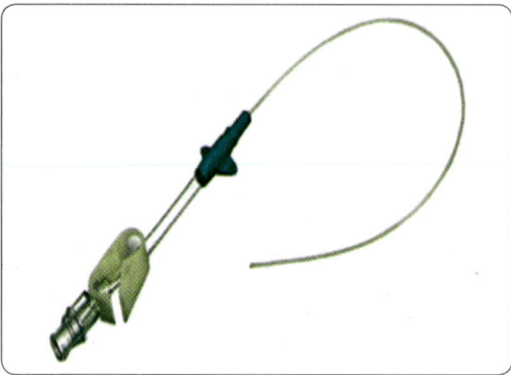

FIG. 1: Single lumen catheter

❑ Multi-lumen catheter (Fig. 2)

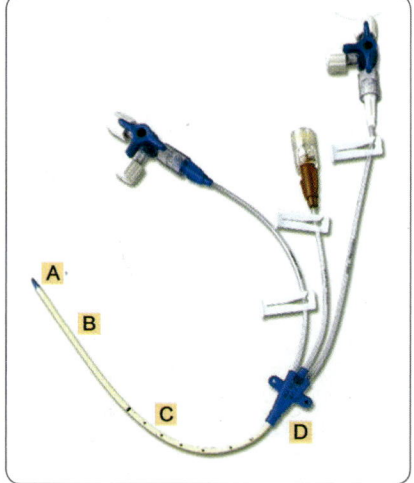

FIG. 2: Multi-lumen catheter

CENTRAL VENOUS CATHETER INSERTION SITES

Commonly used sites are:

❑ Subclavian vein

❑ Jugular vein

Other potential sites are:

❑ Brachial vein

❑ Median and Basilic vein

❑ Femoral vein

PREPARATION OF ARTICLES AND THEIR PURPOSES

Articles	Purposes
❏ Sterile pack of containing swabs, gallipots, kidney tray	
❏ Sterile gloves, gown and mask	
❏ Local anesthetic agent (1% lidocaine)	
❏ 10 mL syringe	❏ To give anesthesia
❏ 20 mL syringe	❏ To aspirate and flush the light

Purposes

- ❏ To administer medication, especially injection dopamine.
- ❏ To provide parenteral nutrition
- ❏ To have intravenous access for long time
- ❏ To measure central venous pressure.
- ❏ To administer large amount of fluid in short duration.

Indications

- ❏ Monitor central venous pressure (CVP)
- ❏ Large-bore intravenous access
- ❏ Rapid fluid resuscitation
- ❏ Rapid administration of blood replacement therapy
- ❏ Infusion of therapeutic drugs
- ❏ Administration of chemotherapy and vasoactive substances
- ❏ Renal dialysis
- ❏ Aspiration of air embolism
- ❏ Other substances which are harmful through subcutaneous or peripheral vascular route

Contraindications

- ❏ Uncooperative patient
- ❏ Infection at the insertion site
- ❏ Coagulopathy
- ❏ Systemic infection
- ❏ Presence of indwelling catheters or pacing wires at the insertion site
- ❏ The affected side in case of mastectomy
- ❏ Obstructed veins

STEPS OF PROCEDURE AND RATIONALE

Steps	Rationale
❏ Explain the procedure to the patient	❏ To gain patient's cooperation and reduce anxiety
❏ Obtain written consent	❏ Prevent legal risk
❏ Provide privacy	❏ To make patient more comfortable.
❏ Assemble articles at the bedside	❏ Avoid inconvenience during procedure. Save time and energy

Contd…

Assisting in Insertion of Central Venous Catheter

Steps	Rationale
❑ Position the patient to lie flat with slight head down. Turn head to the left and slightly up	❑ Identify the site for catheter insertion
❑ Wash hands thoroughly and don the gloves	❑ Prevent cross infection
❑ Assist physician in cleaning this site with Betadine, spirit and administration of local anesthesia	❑ It helps to create sterile field and minimize contamination. Reduces pain sensation of the patient
❑ Attach 10 mL syringe to the needle and assist physician in inserting the needle into selected vein	
❑ Once the needle is within the lumen of the vein remove the syringe and insert guidewire in the needle	
❑ Once the wire is positioned, the physician withdraws the needle. Provide scalpel blade to the physician to make a small nick in the skin over the guidewire	❑ Small nick on the skin allows insertion of dilating device
❑ Assist by holding the patient's head steadily while dilating device is pass down the wire and insert it fully	❑ For easy insertion
❑ Physician removes the dilating device and guidewire and confirms the position by aspirating blood from the catheter	❑ Confirm the position of needle
❑ Provide sterile normal saline to flush the catheter to keep the lumen patent	❑ Prevent clogging of catheter lumen
❑ Assist to secure the catheter in place	❑ Prevent displacement
❑ Provide three-way to the physician to attach it with the lumen. Ensure that every port is flushed	❑ Three way provides more excess
❑ Assist in applying the dressing over the catheter insertion site	❑ Dressing minimizes chances of infection
❑ Provide comfortable position to the patient	
❑ Discard waste materials, clean and replace the articles	❑ To prevent infection and prepare for next use
❑ Record the procedure in nurse's notes with proper time, date, type of catheter, insertion site and response of client	❑ Helps to communicate information to health professionals

CHAPTER 17

Central Venous Catheter Care— Change Dressing

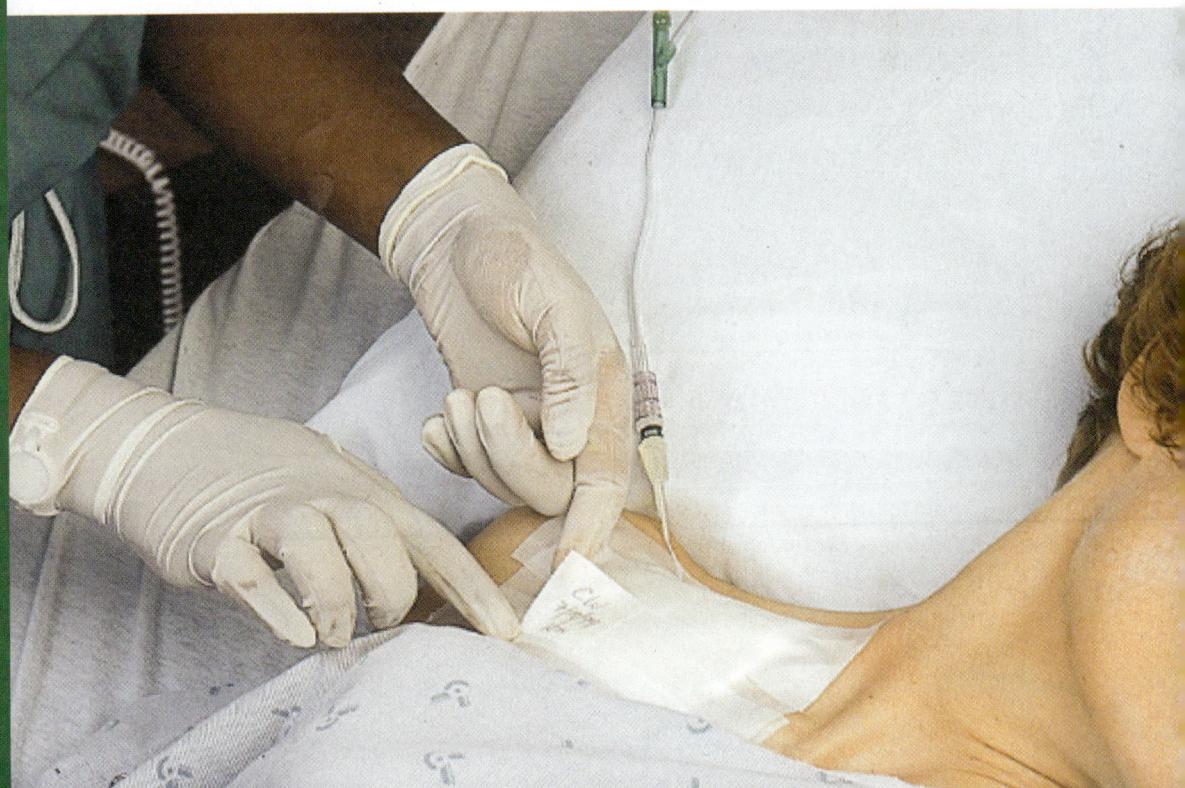

DEFINITION

Provide catheter care by changing dressing at insertion site of central venous catheter. It is done when dressing become loose, wet or at a regular interval as per policy.

PURPOSES

❑ To prevent infection
❑ To maintain hygiene at the site of catheter insertion (Fig. 1).

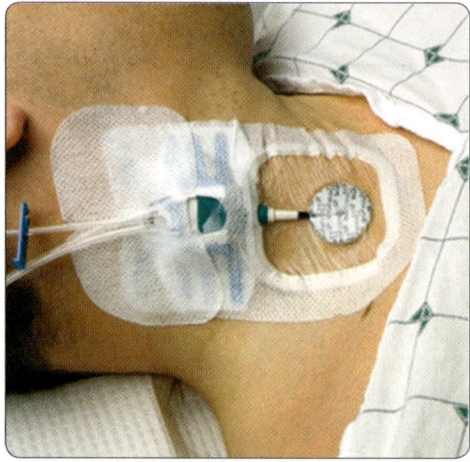

FIG. 1: Maintain hygiene at the site of catheter insertion

PREPARATION OF ARTICLES AND THEIR PURPOSES

Articles	Purposes
A sterile dressing tray containing:	
❑ Thumb forcep-1	❑ To squeeze dipped swabs
❑ Artery forceps-2	❑ To hold cotton swabs and gauze pieces
❑ Cotton swabs and gauze pieces	❑ For cleaning
❑ Gallipot	❑ To pour betadine solution
❑ Sterile gloves	
A clean tray containing: ❑ Clean gloves	❑ To prevent infection
❑ Betadine solutions and spirit	❑ To kill microbes

STEPS OF PROCEDURE AND RATIONALE

Steps	Rationale
❑ Explain the procedure to the patient	❑ To gain patient's cooperation
❑ Perform hand hygiene and don clean gloves	❑ To prevent cross infection
❑ Remove old dressing carefully	❑ To avoid discomfort and pain
❑ Assess insertion site for any redness, tenderness or swelling	❑ To check signs of the infection

Contd…

Steps	Rationale
❏ Remove gloves and put on sterile gloves	❏ To maintain sterility
❏ Clean the site with betadine and spirits swabs in a circular motion about 2–3 cm	❏ To remove microorganisms
❏ Apply betadine ointment at the insertion site if ordered	❏ To reduce growth of bacteria at the insertion site
❏ Cover the dressing with gauze pieces (preferably used transparent dressing)	❏ To prevent bacteria from entering the insertion site
❏ Label the dressing with date and time	❏ To plan for next dressing change
❏ Secure tubing to client's clothing	❏ To prevent dislodging
❏ Remove gloves and discard used material ❏ Clean and replace the articles	❏ To prevent cross infection and keep articles ready for next use
❏ Perform hand hygiene	❏ To prevent infection
❏ Record the procedure on nurse's notes	❏ Proper communication to other health members

NOTES

CHAPTER 18

Assisting in Thoracentesis

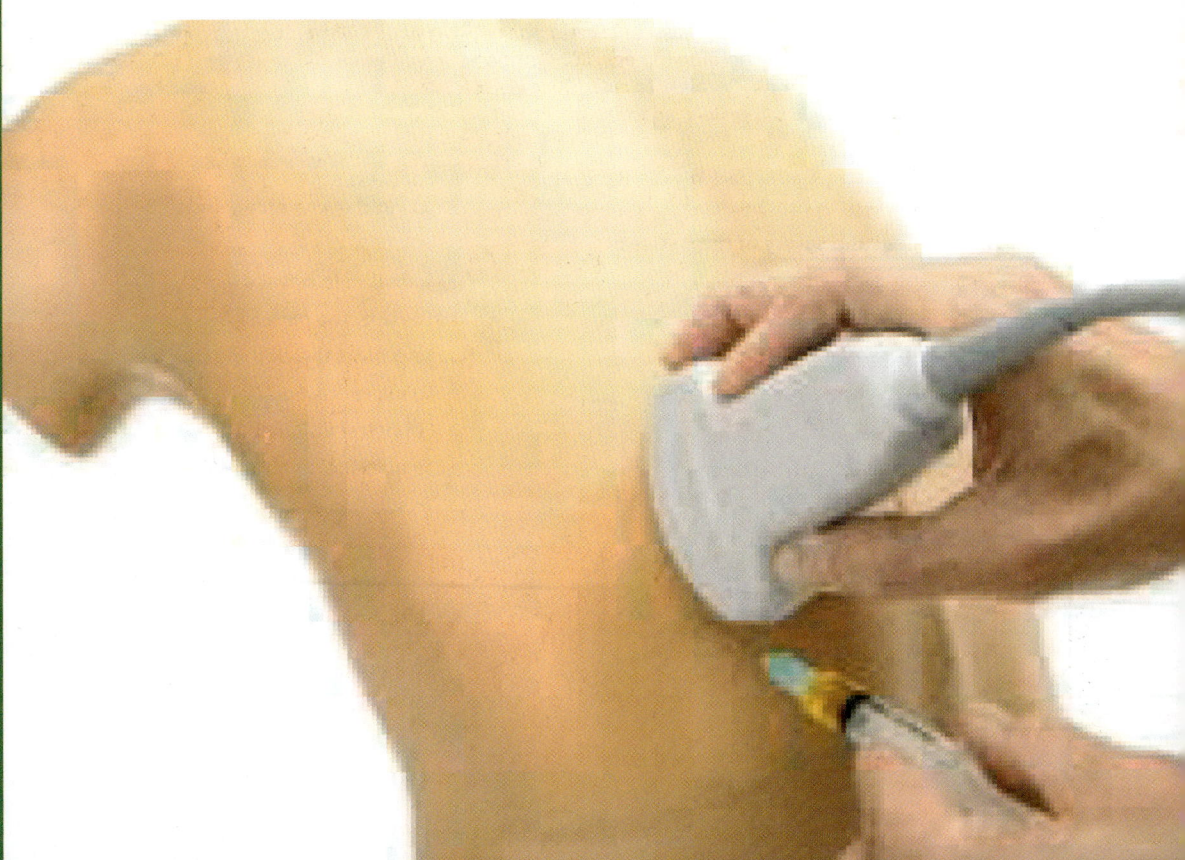

INTRODUCTION

In the pleural space a thin layer of pleural fluid remains normally. A sample of this can be obtained by thoracentesis or by tube thoracotomy.

DEFINITION

Thoracentesis is the aspiration of pleural fluid or air for diagnostic or therapeutic purposes by a doctor with the assistance of a nurse.

PURPOSES

- ❑ Removal of fluid and air from the pleural cavity.
- ❑ Diagnostic aspiration of pleural fluid
- ❑ Pleural biopsy
- ❑ Installation of medication into pleural space.

PREPARATION OF ARTICLES AND THEIR PURPOSES

Articles	Purposes
A. A tray containing:	
❑ Spirit, iodine, tincture benzoin, local anesthetic agent	❑ To maintain aseptic technique ❑ To minimize pain
❑ A cough sedative, mist stimulant and a medicine glass	❑ To suppress cough during procedure
❑ A sterile culture tube	❑ To send the collected specimen for culture
❑ A minor surgical set or sterile tray containing artery forceps, scissors, sponge holding forceps, 2cc syringe with needle, jelco 14 no. Secalen T (18G), 20cc and 50c syringe with a three way adapter, an IV, set. A sterile kidney tray	❑ For doing thoracentesis under the surgical aseptic technique
❑ A sterile dressing, gauze pack gloves, Band-Aid ❑ Cheatle forceps in container	❑ For dressing ❑ To hand over sterile things
B. For comfort and safety of the patient:	
❑ A screen	❑ To maintain privacy
❑ A blanket or a sheet	❑ To cover the patient
❑ A mackintosh with a towel	❑ To protect the clothing from vomitus
❑ A cardiac table or back rest as needed	❑ To make position
❑ Good light	❑ For better visibility
❑ A kidney tray and paper bag	❑ To hold the vomitus
❑ A sputum cup	❑ To spit the sputum
C. For doctor	
❑ A sterile gown, a mask and gloves	❑ To maintain aseptic technique
❑ Scrub up articles	❑ To scrub hands

STEPS OF PROCEDURE AND RATIONALE

Steps	Rationale
❏ Assess the general condition of the patient and take a written consent form	❏ To know base line data and legal requirement
❏ A thorough chest examination is to be done and identify there is any allergy toward medicine	❏ To confirm there is no chest abnormality and any allergic reactions
❏ Explain the procedure to the patient. Explain him clearly about not to move during the procedure	❏ To make the patient comfortable and reduce his anxiety
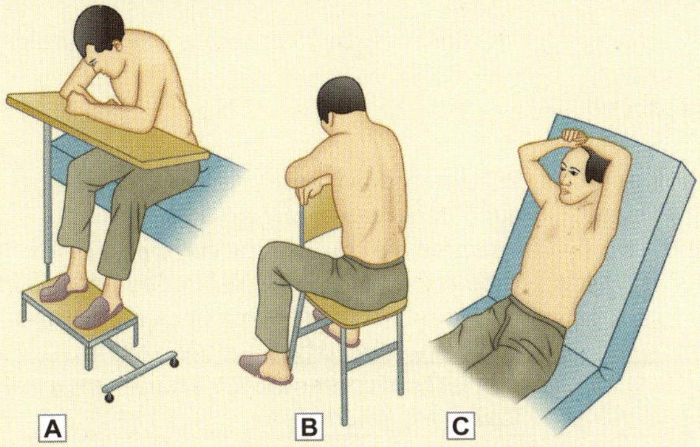 ❏ Provide a comfortable position to the patient. Place the patient in an upright position in one of the following position (Fig. 1) ❏ Sitting on the edge of the bed with feet supported and arms and head on a padded bed table 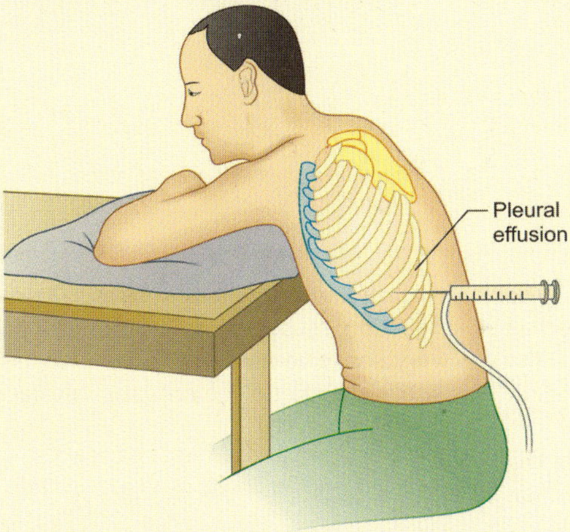	❏ These positions facilitate the removal of fluid that usually localizes at the lower part of the chest

Pleural effusion

FIG. 1: Position for the thoracentesis

❏ Make the patient to sit on a chair with arms and head resting on the back of the chair
❏ Elevate the bed 30°–45° and make the patient to lie on the unaffected side if unable to assume a sitting position

Three different comfortable positions of the patient is depicted below in Figs 2A to C:

FIGS 2A TO C: Three different comfortable positions of the patient for thoracentesis

Contd…

Assisting in Thoracentesis

Steps	Rationale
❏ Support and reassure the patient during the procedure ❏ Apply cold application ice packs at the insertion site to get the anesthetic effect or local anesthesia ❏ Advise the patient not to cough during the procedure	❏ To reduce pain, unexpected movement by the patient ❏ It causes trauma to the visceral pleura and lungs
❏ Expose the entire chest so that the site of aspiration can be determined easily. 　○ Examine the chest X-ray film properly (Fig. 3) **FIG. 3:** Chest X-ray 　○ Chest Percussion	❏ If the thoracentesisis due to accumulation of fluid the site for insertion is seventh intercostal space. ❏ If it is due to air in the pleural cavity the thoracentesis site is in the second or third intercostals space in the midclavicular line.
❏ The doctor under aseptic condition performs the procedure. After the skin is cleaned the physician injects a local anesthetic agent with a small caliber needle into the intercostals space	❏ An intradermal wheal is raised slowly rapid injection causes pain. The parietal pleura is very sensitive and should be well-infiltrated with anesthetic before the thoracentesis needle is passed
❏ The physician advances the thoracentesis needle with the syringe attached. When the pleural place is reached suction may be applied with a syringe	
❏ A 20 mL syringe with a three adapter is attached to the needle. One end of the adapter is attached to the needle and the other top the tubing leading to a receptacle that receives the fluid being aspirated	❏ When a large quantity of fluid is withdrawn, a three way adapter serves to keep air entering the pleural cavity
❏ After the needle is withdrawn, pressure is applied over the puncture site and a small sterile dressing is applied.	❏ To cover the wound
❏ The patient is placed on bed rest and a chest X-ray is taken after thoracentesis	❏ Chest X-ray verifies that there is no pneumothorax
❏ Record the total amount of fluid, its color and its viscosity. If requested, prepare a sample of fluid for laboratory evaluation. A specimen container with formalin is required if pleural biopsy is sent	❏ The fluid may be clear serous blood purulent, etc.
❏ Evaluate the patient at intervals for increasing respiratory rate, faintness, vertigo, tightness in chest, uncontrollable cough, blood tinged, frothy mucus, a rapid pulse and a sign of hypoxemia	❏ Pneumothorax, tension pneumothorax, subcutaneous emphysema pyogenic infection are some of the complication of thoracocentesis. Other serious complications end as pulmonary edema or cardiac distress can be produced by a sudden shift in mediastinal content when a large amount of fluid is aspirated

COMPLICATIONS

- ❑ Pneumothorax
- ❑ Subcutaneous emphysema
- ❑ Pyogenic infection
- ❑ Pulmonary edema
- ❑ Cardiac distress

Points to Remember

- ❑ Observe a strict aseptic technique during the procedure.
- ❑ Closely watch the patient after the procedure for 2–3 hours.
- ❑ Do not allow the patient to cough during the procedure to avoid injury to the lungs.

NOTES

CHAPTER 19

Abdominal
Paracentesis

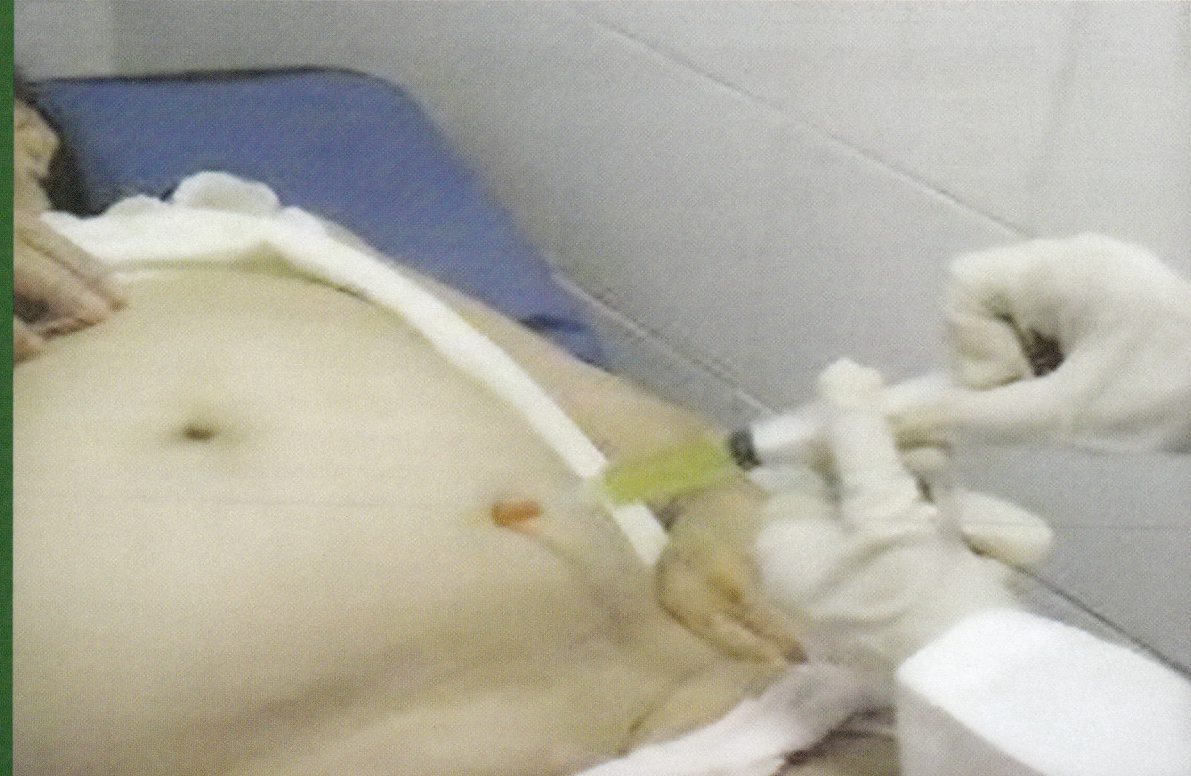

DEFINITION

Abdominal paracentesis (Fig. 1) is the removal of fluid from peritoneal cavity or abdominal cavity. It is also called peritoneal tap.

PURPOSES

- ❑ For diagnostic purpose
- ❑ For therapeutic purpose to relieve pressure on abdominal cavity and pleural cavity
- ❑ To prepare for other procedures

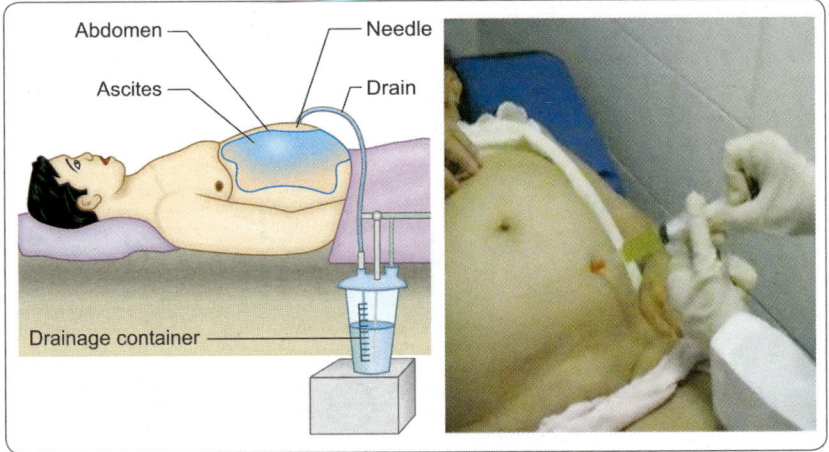

FIG. 1: Abdominal paracentesis

ARTICLES REQUIRED AND THEIR PURPOSES

Articles	Purposes
A covered sterile tray containing: ❑ 2 mL syringe –1 ❑ 25G X1" Needle –2 ❑ 23G.X1 ¼ Needle –1 ❑ Small bowls–2	❑ To administer local anesthetic
❑ 5" dissecting forceps or sponge holder–1 ❑ Cotton balls–6 ❑ Gauze pads–2	❑ To clean the skin
❑ Scalpel–1 ❑ Trocar and cannula–1	❑ To make incision to insert into abdominal cavity and to drain out fluid
❑ Pint pressure–1	❑ To measure the abdominal fluid
❑ Fenestrated towel–1	❑ To cover the area and to maintain sterile field and to expose only the require path

Contd…

Articles	Purposes
❑ Surgical drape ❑ 12" rubber tubing–1 ❑ Screw clamp–1 ❑ A skin preparation tray ❑ A sterile surgical towel ❑ A dressing set ❑ A bowl of warm water ❑ Razor set with blade ❑ A bowl of 6 cotton balls ❑ 6 gauze squares ❑ A soap dish with soap ❑ Savlon1:30 in a bottle ❑ Torch	❑ To prepare the skin and disinfect the local area for a sterile procedure ❑ To prepare the skin
❑ A kidney tray ❑ A mackintosh ❑ A treatment towel ❑ A paper bag	❑ To protect bed linen and discard waste
❑ Basin ❑ Sponge cloths ❑ Jugs–2 ❑ Buckets–2	❑ For cleaning
❑ Sterile gloves–1 pair ❑ A sterile gauze mask ❑ Local anesthetic	❑ To keep the hand sterile by using gloves ❑ To anesthetize the part
❑ Sterile specimen bottles-3	❑ To collect specimen
❑ Many tailed binder-1 ❑ Safety pin-1 ❑ Back rest-1	❑ To provide abdominal comfort ❑ To secure the binder ❑ To give a propped up position
❑ Spirit, iodine, Tr. Benzoin, sponge holding forceps, gauze pieces ❑ A screen	❑ To prepare the sterile field ❑ To clean the part ❑ To maintain privacy

CARE BEFORE PROCEDURE AND RATIONALE

Steps	Rationale
❑ Assemble equipment and bring to the bedside.	❑ To save time, energy and material
❑ Explain the procedure to the patient	❑ To prevent fear and to gain confidence
❑ Ask the patient to void or catheterize if necessary	❑ To prevent injury to the bladder
❑ Follow strict aseptic techniques during the procedure	❑ To prevent cross infection
❑ Keep the patient warm and comfortable	❑ To prevent peripheral vasoconstriction and shock
❑ Keep drugs and equipment ready to treat shock	❑ Shock is one of the complications so the drugs should be kept ready
❑ Take consent	❑ To have legal safety
❑ Place the screen	❑ To maintain privacy
❑ Prepare the skin, i.e. from nipple line to pelvis. In female below the breast	❑ To prevent infection

Contd…

Abdominal Paracentesis

Steps	Rationale
❑ Record vital signs	❑ To identify shock and to treat it at an early stage. Sudden withdrawal of abdominal fluid which may cause shock
❑ Change the client's garments and put on a loose gown and pin up the gown during the procedure	❑ To prevent inconvenient interference with the procedure. Help to keep clean and prevent cross infection

CARE DURING THE PROCEDURE AND RATIONALE

Steps	Rationale
❑ Fanfold the top linen down to the pubic area	❑ To expose the area and prevent interference
❑ Expose the area below the nipple up to the pubic area	❑ To minimize exposure of the patient and keep him warm
❑ Place the bucket in position to receive the abdominal fluid	❑ To prevent spillage and have accurate measurement
❑ Place the client in Fowler's position	❑ Comfortable for the client and full expansion of thoracic cavity
❑ Place mackintosh	❑ To protect bed linen
❑ Wash hands and open the sterile tray	❑ To prevent cross infection
❑ Open the dressing set and take forceps and hand over the surgical towel from the sterile tray to the doctor for wiping hands	❑ To assist the physician and avoid cross infection
❑ Assist the doctor in drawing local anesthetic. After infiltration of the area with local anesthetic the doctor will insert trocar and cannula half way between umbilicus and anterior superior iliac spine	❑ To anesthetize the site of paracentesis. Local anesthetic local pain due to the procedure to anesthetize the site of paracentesis.
❑ Trocar is removed by the doctor and a rubber tubing is attached to the cannula to drain out fluid	❑ To drain out the abdominal fluid
❑ Place the rubber tubing in a sterile pint measure and adjust the rate of flow with a screw clamp	❑ Helps in measuring the drained out fluid and prevents cross infection. Provides a sterile field and prevent ascending infection
❑ If specimens are to be sent collect the abdominal fluid in the specified sample bottles	❑ For diagnostic purpose
❑ When the desired amount of fluid is removed then procedure has to be discontinued. Place the gauze piece and gauze pads after cleaning with sterile cotton swab over the wound.	❑ To prevent leakage of abdominal fluid. To protect the wound
❑ Apply any tailed bandage over the abdomen	❑ To prevent shock and collapse. To maintain intra-abdominal pressure
❑ Place the client in a comfortable position in the bed check pulse and BP	❑ To make the patient comfortable and check any untoward signs and symptoms

CARE AFTER THE PROCEDURE AND RATIONALE

Steps	Rationale
❑ The equipment to be removed from bedside, tidy up the unit after making the client comfortable	❑ For neatness and to clean the equipment
❑ If the abdominal fluid is collected in a bucket measure accurately with a pint measure note the characteristics of fluid and record	❑ To measure accurately ❑ To know the amount, color and consistency of fluid
❑ Wash, dry and replace the equipment	❑ To prevent cross infection
❑ Check the vital signs every ½ hour for 2 hours every ½ hour for 4 hours and every 4 hours for 24 hours	❑ To detect shock in early stages and treat
❑ Observe the dressing for excessive soakage	❑ As there is incision abdominal fluid may leak
❑ Observe for: ❑ Complications, hypovolemia, collapse ❑ Infection and peritonitis ❑ Injury to blood vessels and other abdominal organs ❑ Renal failure due to systemic circulation	❑ There are complications which are possible. So the complications need to be detected and treated at an early stage
❑ Record the time of procedure with vital signs and any complications in the nurse's notes and inform the doctor	❑ Helps to communicate information to health professionals

AFTER CARE

❑ Observe the patient for 30 minutes for the signs of hypertension, bleeding or abdominal distress.
❑ Provide postprocedure analgesics.

CONTRAINDICATIONS

❑ Marked bowel distension
❑ Previous abdominal surgery
❑ Patient is on anticoagulation
❑ Infected abdominal wall

Points to Remember

❑ Patient is advised to take rest postprocedure.
❑ Remove the dressing after 24 hours.

Abdominal Paracentesis

NOTES

CHAPTER 20

Care of the Patient with Chest Drainage

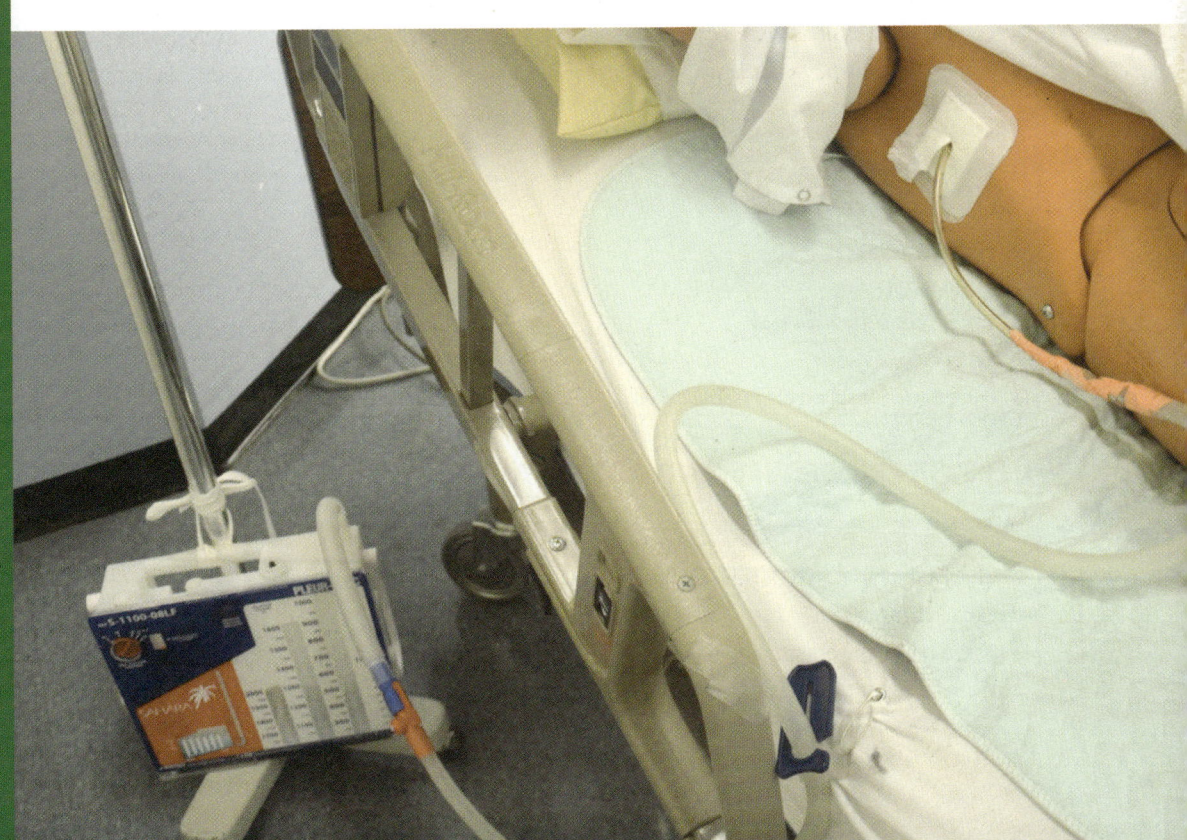

DEFINITION

Intercostal water seal drainage system is insertion of tubes into the pleural cavity with attached drainage system to remove air, blood, or fluid from the pleural cavity.

PURPOSES

❑ To drain fluid from thoracic cavity
❑ To promote re-expansion of lungs

INDICATIONS

❑ Pneumothorax
❑ Hemothorax
❑ Thoracotomy
❑ Chest surgery
❑ Chest trauma
❑ Pleural effusion
❑ Chylothorax
❑ Postoperative cardiac disease

ARTICLES REQUIRED AND THEIR PURPOSES

Articles	Purposes
❑ Clean trolley	❑ To arrange the clean articles
❑ Chest drainage bottle holder	❑ To hold the drainage bottle
❑ Long and short tubes (plastic/glass)	❑ To drain fluid or air into the bottle
❑ Sterile chest drainage bottle with two-way or three-way cork	❑ To collect the air or fluid drain from the chest
❑ Sterile water or sterile normal saline	❑ To know the amount of air expelled out
❑ Sterile pint measure	❑ To measure the amount of blood
❑ Clean clamps -2 no	❑ To clamp the flow of air or blood
❑ Sterile gloves	❑ To prevent cross infection
❑ Clean mask	❑ To prevent yourself from infection
❑ Water proof adhesive tape	❑ To place the chest tube in position
❑ Scissors	
❑ Receptacle for soiled disposable items	

STEPS OF PROCEDURE AND RATIONALE

Steps	Rationale
❑ Check the physician order and nursing care plan for specific instructions	
❑ Explain the procedure to the patient and relatives	❑ To get patient's cooperation
❑ Assemble all the equipment near the bedside	❑ It saves time and energy
❑ Wash hands and wear sterile gloves	

Contd…

Principles and Procedures of NURSING FOUNDATIONS

Steps	Rationale

- ❑ Prepare chest drainage bottle

For one bottle (Fig. 1):
- ❑ Open a sterile two-way bottle and add sterile water
- ❑ Ensure that the distal end of the long tube immersed in 2–3 cm of water
- ❑ Mark the water level in the bottle
- ❑ Insert long- and short-tubes through the two-way cork into the bottle

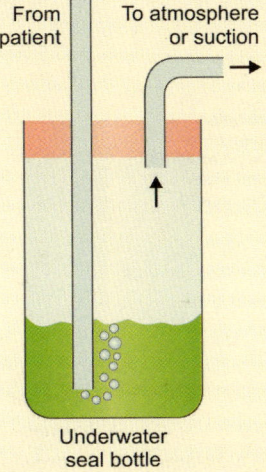

FIG. 1: One bottle system for chest drainage

For two-bottle system (Fig. 2):
- ❑ In case of two-bottle system the first bottle is used to collect fluid and air from pleural space and the second serves as water seal chamber.

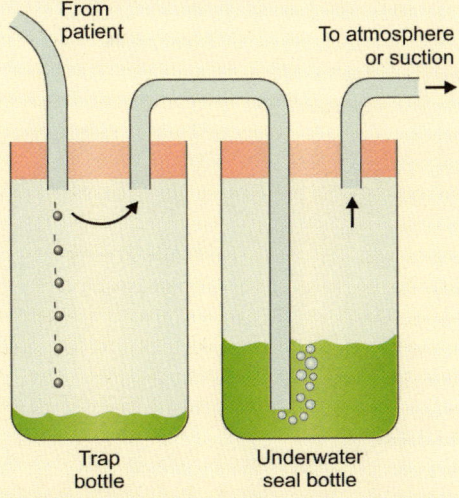

FIG. 2: Two-bottle system for chest drainage

Three-bottle system (Fig. 3):
- ❑ In case of three-bottle system the first bottle is used to collect fluid and air from pleural space, second bottle serves as water seal and the third bottle is to control the amount of suction applied.

Contd...

Care of the Patient with Chest Drainage

Steps	Rationale
❑ Prepare the first and second bottles as in two-bottle system ❑ Add 20 cm of sterile water in the third sterile bottle. ❑ Connect the bottles 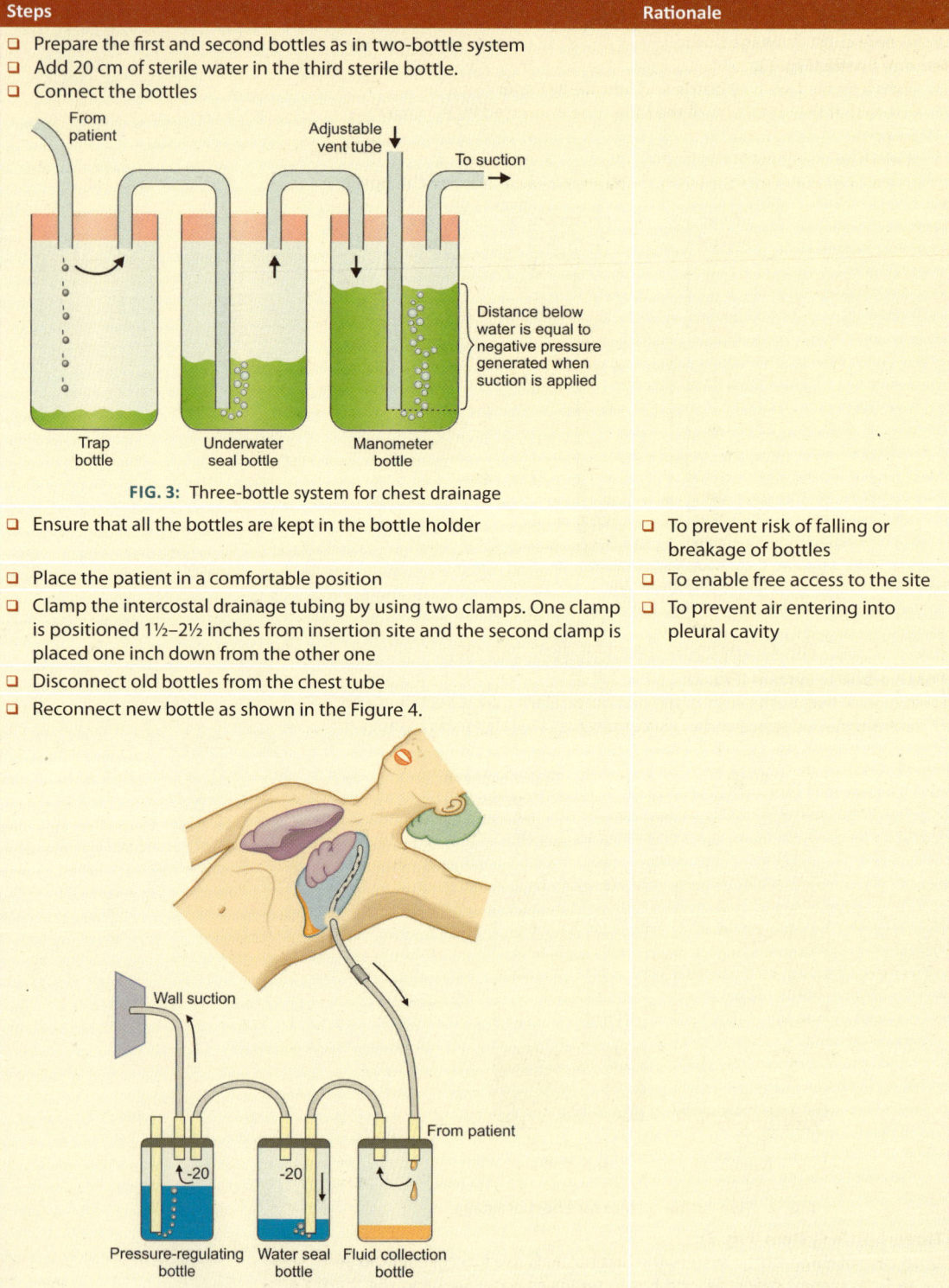 **FIG. 3:** Three-bottle system for chest drainage	
❑ Ensure that all the bottles are kept in the bottle holder	❑ To prevent risk of falling or breakage of bottles
❑ Place the patient in a comfortable position	❑ To enable free access to the site
❑ Clamp the intercostal drainage tubing by using two clamps. One clamp is positioned 1½–2½ inches from insertion site and the second clamp is placed one inch down from the other one	❑ To prevent air entering into pleural cavity
❑ Disconnect old bottles from the chest tube ❑ Reconnect new bottle as shown in the Figure 4.	

FIG. 4: Left-sided pneumothorax

Contd…

Principles and Procedures of NURSING FOUNDATIONS

Steps	Rationale
❏ Keep the bottle 0.5–1 m below the chest of the patient	❏ To prevent water being sucked into the chest
❏ Release the clamps from the chest tube	❏ Prolonged clamping may lead to develop tension pneumothorax
❏ See for repeated fluctuation in the water level in the distal end of chest tube	❏ These fluctuations correspond to the patient's breathing and indicate that the system is patent ❏ Absence of fluctuation indicates that the chest tube is blocked or the lungs are expanded. This can be confirmed by percussion, auscultation and chest radiography
❏ Position the patient comfortably on the bed	
❏ Wash and dry hands	❏ Prevents transmission
❏ Record the procedure	❏ Acts as communication among staff
❏ Continue monitoring the patient	❏ Helps to know response to new system

COMPLICATIONS

❏ Pneumothorax
❏ Bleeding at the drain site
❏ Infection of insertion site
❏ Accidental disconnection of system
❏ Accidental drain removal
❏ Unable to remove chest drainage
❏ Retained drain during removal

Points to Remember

❏ Fluctuation in the tubing should be there according to respiration of the patient.
❏ All the three bottles should be air tight. No leakage of air.

Care of the Patient with Chest Drainage

NOTES

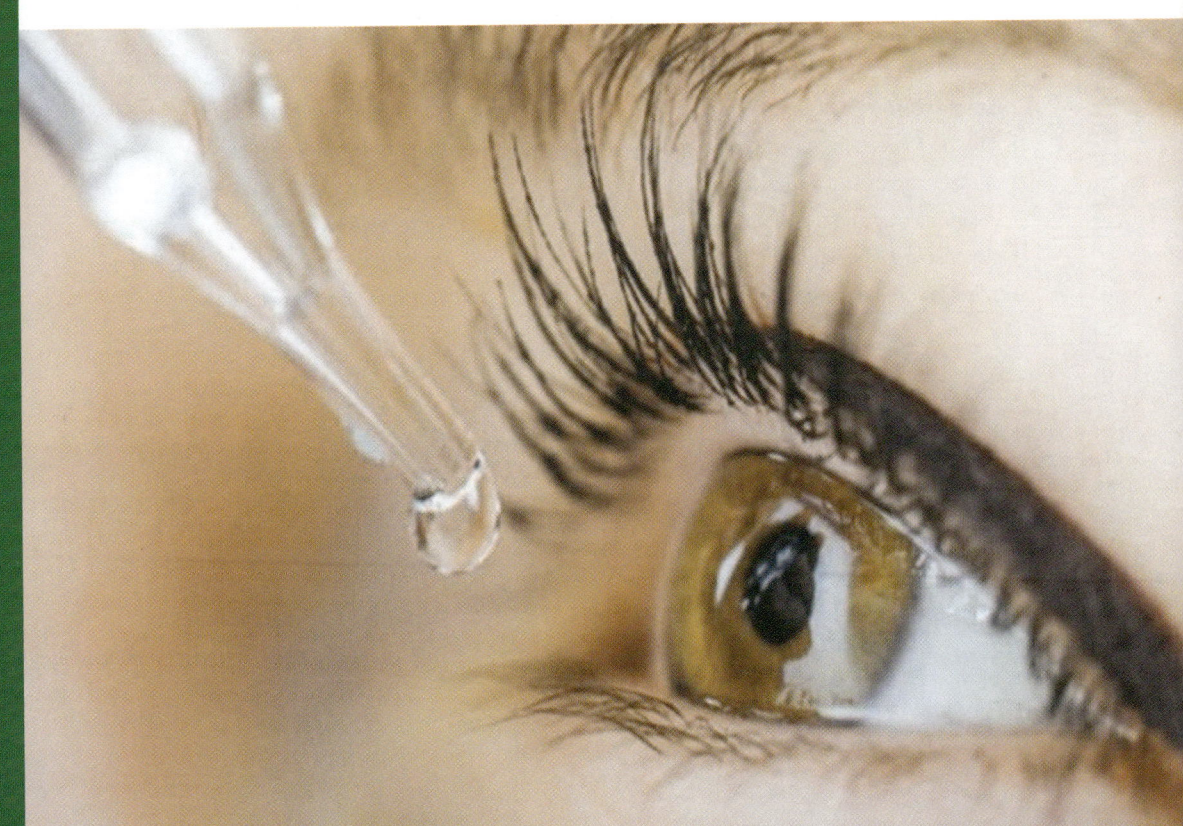

CHAPTER 21

Eye Irrigation

DEFINITION

Eye irrigation is the washing of the conjunctival sac with a solution.

PURPOSES

- ❑ To clean and remove secretions
- ❑ To relieve inflammation, congestion and pain
- ❑ To relieve foreign bodies
- ❑ To apply medication for antiseptic effect
- ❑ For thermal effects

SOLUTIONS USED

- ❑ Plain water
- ❑ Normal saline
- ❑ Boric acid 2%
- ❑ Silver nitrate 1%
- ❑ Acriflavine 1%

ARTICLES REQUIRED AND THEIR PURPOSES

Articles	Purposes
❑ A tray containing: ○ An eye dropper, a syringe or plastic bottle with the prescribed solutions and an IV set with attached tubing or a sterile irrigation can with tubing	❑ To irrigate the eye
❑ A bowl or jug with a solution ordered	❑ To irrigate the eye
❑ Sterile wet swab in a bowl	❑ To clean eye before the procedure
❑ Sterile cotton bowls and a small towel	❑ To dry the eye after the procedure
❑ Thumb forceps in boiled cold water	❑ To handle sterile articles
❑ A mackintosh and a towel	❑ To protect bed from soiling
❑ A kidney tray and a paper bag	❑ To receive waste
❑ An IV stand if needed	❑ To hold the begs of fluid/medicine
❑ Medication if ordered	❑ As prescribed for the patient

STEPS OF PROCEDURE AND RATIONALE

Steps	Rationale
❑ Explain the procedure to the patient and instruct him to tilt his head toward the side of the affected side of the eye. The patient should sit or lie in a supine position	❑ To win the patient's confidence and cooperation
❑ Place the mackintosh and towel under the head	❑ To protect the linen from soiling
❑ The kidney tray should be placed at the affected side of the face with convex side near the eye to receive the outflow	❑ To protect the bed/cloths from soiling

Contd…

Steps	Rationale
❑ Wash hands	❑ To prevent transfer of microorganism
❑ Clean eyelids and eye lashes from the inner canthus to the outer canthus using sterile wet swabs (one on each stroke) without touching the part which will come in contact with the eye	❑ Any crust on the eye lids and lashes should be washed off before irrigation
❑ Irrigate the eye using the irrigator ❑ Adjust the flow of the liquid by adjusting the height of the irrigator ○ Test the temperature of the irrigating solution (98–100°F) by pouring some of the fluid on back of your hand and ask the client to close the eye and pour a little solution on eyelids	❑ To prevent burns
❑ Evert the lower conjunctival sac (pull down the lower lid with the index finger) instruct the patient to look up avoid touching the eye with nozzle held 2 cm above the eye	❑ To prevent injury to sensitive cornea
❑ Allow irrigating fluid to flow from the inner canthus to the outer canthus, ask the patient to look up while irrigating	❑ To prevent infection of the nasolacrimal duct
❑ Irrigate the eye till the desired effect is achieved	❑ For proper cleaning of the eye
❑ Repeat the procedure on the other side if necessary. Separate articles and solutions should be used for the other eye if needed	❑ To avoid the spread of infection from one eye to another
❑ Dry the face with sterile small towel/dry swab	❑ To provide comfort
❑ Record the type and amount of fluid used as well as the effectiveness	❑ Provide documentation of nursing action
❑ Discard the swab and replace all the articles	❑ To keep equipment for next use

COMPLICATIONS

- ❑ Eye injury
- ❑ Corneal scarring
- ❑ Post-traumatic glaucoma
- ❑ Iridodialysis

Point to Remember

❑ This procedure is there for only one eye. Repeat the procedure for another eye.

NOTES

CHAPTER 22

Ear Irrigation

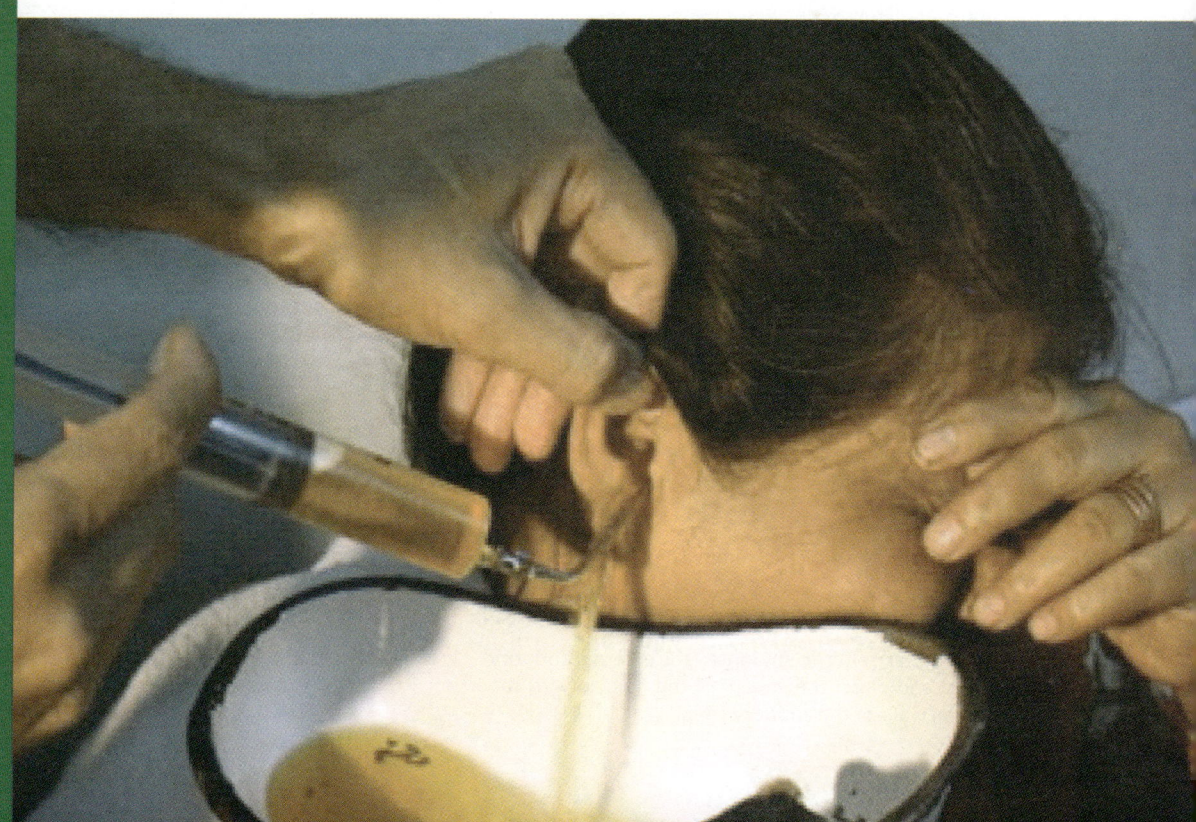

DEFINITION

Ear irrigation is the washing of the external auditory canal with a solution. It is a routine procedure used to remove its excess ear wax and foreign materials from the ear.

PURPOSES

- ❑ To clean the auditory canal
- ❑ To apply heat or cold to the ear
- ❑ To remove any foreign object
- ❑ To relieve pain

SOLUTIONS USED

- ❑ Boric acid 2–4%
- ❑ Sodium bicarbonate solution 1%
- ❑ Normal saline
- ❑ Hydrogen peroxide 2%
- ❑ Plain warm water

ARTICLES REQUIRED AND THEIR PURPOSES

Articles	Purposes
A tray containing:	
❑ An irrigating solution in a sterile container	❑ To irrigate ear
❑ Sterile cotton balls and cotton tipped applicators and a small towel	❑ To clean the external auditory canal
❑ A mackintosh and a towel	❑ To protect the soiling of the bed
❑ A kidney tray and a paper bag	❑ To receive waste
❑ Thumb forceps in a sterile solutions	❑ To transfer sterile articles
❑ An IV stand	❑ To adjust the height of the irrigator

STEPS OF PROCEDURE AND RATIONALE

Steps	Rationale
❑ Explain the procedure and place the patient in a sitting position or dorsal recumbent with his head tilt toward the affected area	❑ To relieve the patient anxiety and gain his cooperation
❑ Spread the mackintosh or towel and put the kidney tray close to the head and under the ear	❑ To receive the irrigating solution and to prevent soiling of bed and clothes
❑ Wash hands	❑ To prevent transfer of microorganism
❑ Use a cloth swab stick to remove any discharge	❑ To prevent carrying discharge deeper into the canal
❑ Test temperature of the solution by pouring at the back of the nurse hand and pinna of the ear	❑ Extreme temperature causes vertigo
❑ Pull the ear gently to straighten the external auditory canal and direct the stream of the fluid toward the lateral walls of the auditory canal	❑ It allows fluid to reach up to tympanic membrane

Contd…

Steps	Rationale
❏ Observe signs of pain and vertigo	
❏ Irrigate the ear till the desired effect is achieved by a steady and continuous flow of the solution	❏ To achieve the desired result
❏ Dry pinna of the ear by using a small towel	❏ To feel comfortable
❏ Remove soiled articles and make the patient comfortable. Instruct the patient to lie on the irrigated side for a few minutes after the procedure	❏ To allow the remaining solutions to drain out of the auditory canal to make the patient relaxed
❏ Record the time of irrigation, kind and amount of the solution, nature of the return flow and effect of the treatment	❏ Documentation of the nursing actions

COMPLICATIONS

❏ Temporary dizziness
❏ Ear canal discomfort or pain
❏ Tinnitus or ringing in the ear

Point to Remember

❏ Ear pain and discomfort is short-lasting, if it is there for one or two days take an appointment and see the doctor.

Ear Irrigation

NOTES

CHAPTER 23

Assisting in Endotracheal Tube Intubation

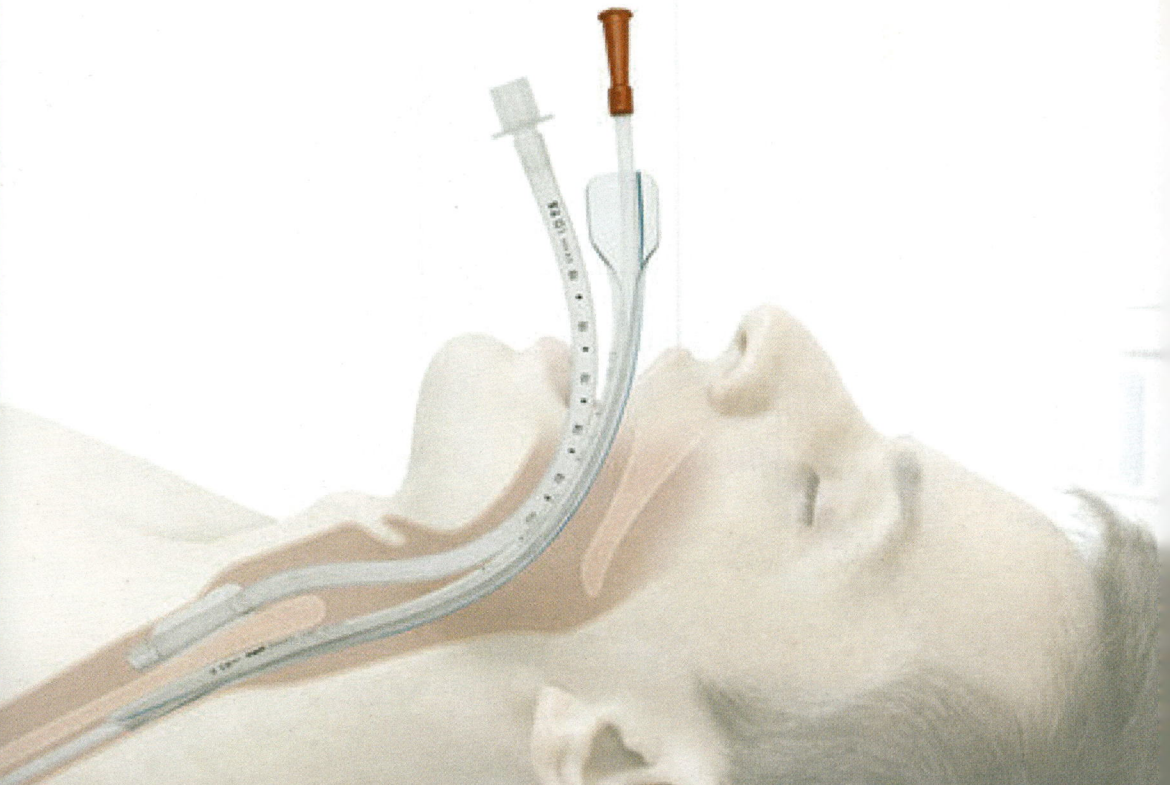

DEFINITION

Assisting in introduction of a hollow plastic tube into the trachea through nose or mouth using aseptic technique to facilitate artificial ventilation and resuscitation (Fig. 1).

PURPOSES

- ❑ To maintain patent airway
- ❑ To ensure adequate oxygen to the patient
- ❑ To provide ventilator assistance whenever required
- ❑ To treat acute respiratory failure.

INDICATIONS

- ❑ Neuromuscular diseases
- ❑ Chest wall injuries
- ❑ Upper airway obstruction
- ❑ Anticipated upper airway obstruction
- ❑ Aspiration prophylaxis
- ❑ Fracture of cervical vertebrae
- ❑ Central nervous system (CNS) depression

ARTICLES REQUIRED AND THEIR PURPOSES

Articles	Purposes
❑ Oxygen source and tubing	❑ To provide oxygen after tube insertion
❑ Suction apparatus with tubing	❑ To clear any secretions
❑ Suction catheter	❑ To clear the secretions
❑ Laryngoscope with appropriate size blade	❑ To visualize the correct place of insertion of tube by seeing uvula
❑ Stiletto	❑ It helps in insertion of tube
❑ Xylocaine gel	❑ To reduce pain while inserting the tube
❑ Oral airway	❑ To provide oxygen source
❑ Disposable syringe 10 mL	❑ For inflating the ET tube and keeps in position
❑ Cotton tape and dynaplast	
❑ Magill forceps	
❑ Sand bag or towel	❑ It supports to extend the neck

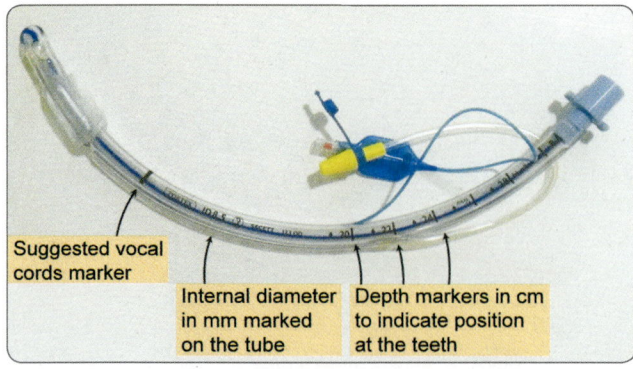

Suggested vocal cords marker

Internal diameter in mm marked on the tube

Depth markers in cm to indicate position at the teeth

FIG. 1: Endotracheal tube

STEPS OF PROCEDURE AND RATIONALE

Steps	Rationale
❑ Explain the procedure to the patient if conscious and get consent from the patient and relatives	❑ Promotes acceptance of procedure and cooperation for procedure from patient
❑ Place the patient in supine position with head extended by keeping sand bag or towel roll under the neck	❑ Promotes access to trachea
❑ Check for loose teeth/dentures or foreign body in throat if it is there remove it with magill forceps	❑ Avoid danger of loose teeth or foreign body causing airway obstruction
❑ Mouth and nose to be sealed with mask Ambu-bag and initiate bagging with oxygen	
❑ Provide laryngoscope to doctor	
❑ Suction the oral cavity	❑ Provides a clear field of work and prevents aspiration when performing oral tracheal insertion
❑ Provide lubricated endotracheal tube with stylet	❑ Helps in insertion of endotracheal tube without chances of injury
❑ Press cricothyroid cartilage with thumb and index finger against esophagus	
❑ Assist while endotracheal tube is introducing into the trachea and remove stylet. Insert the tube up to the marking given 22 cm marking at the incisor teeth	
❑ Verify placement of tube by auscultation or by listening for airflow through tube and observe bilateral chest movement	❑ To confirm the placement of the tube
❑ Connect Ambu-bag with oxygen attached to endotracheal tube	
❑ Inflate the cuff of the endotracheal tube with 10 mL syringe	❑ To prevent chances of tube displacement and aspiration
❑ Insert an oral airway and apply endotracheal suctioning if necessary	
❑ Endotracheal tube is to be positioned by using adhesive tape	
❑ Connect to the ventilator if needed	

COMPLICATIONS

❑ Laryngeal or tracheal injury
❑ Pulmonary infection and sepsis
❑ Dependence of artificial airway
❑ Laryngospasm

Point to Remember

❑ Always discuss with consultant anesthetist regarding specific patient requirements and inflation pressures for cuffed endotracheal tube.

Assisting in Endotracheal Tube Intubation

NOTES

CHAPTER 24

Assisting with Obtaining a Pap Smear

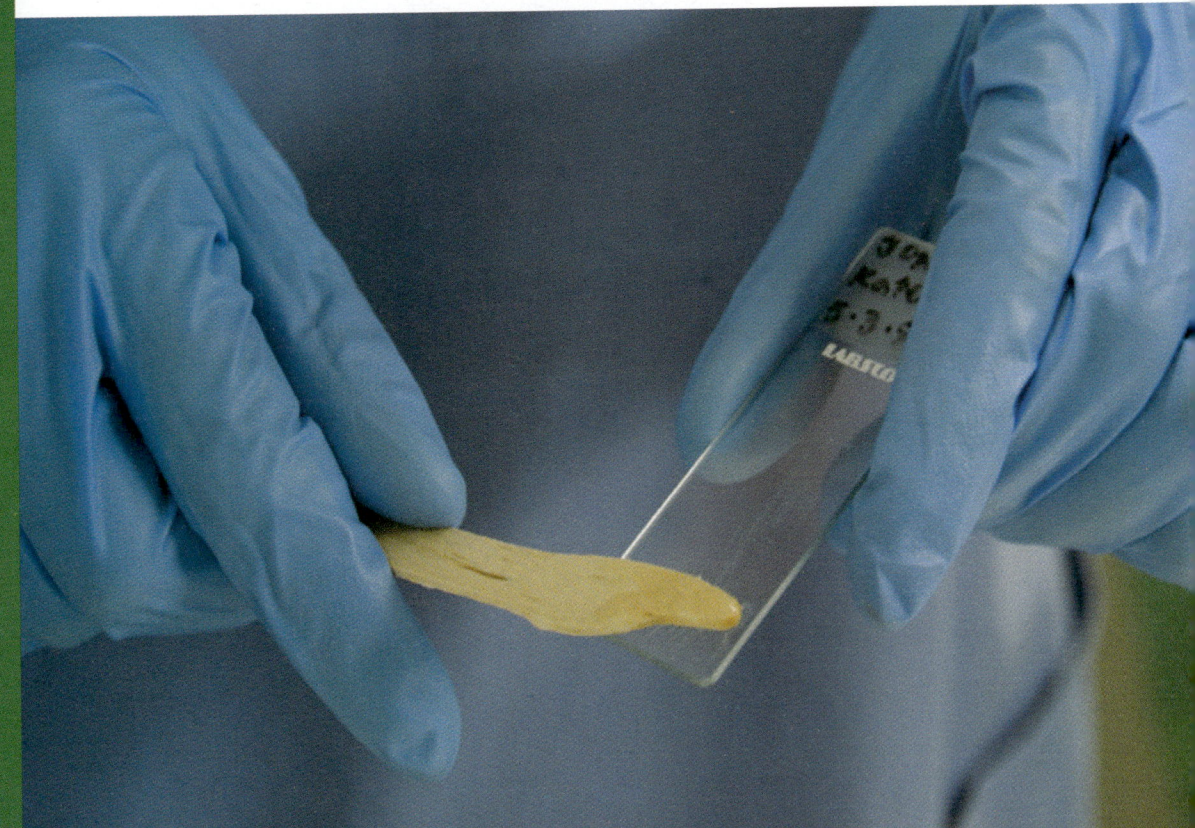

DEFINITION

A Pap smear is also known as Papanicolaou's smear, it is a microscopic examination of cells scraped from the cervix and are used to detect cancerous and precancerous conditions of the cervix and other medical conditions.

PURPOSES

- ❑ To detect cervical and vaginal carcinomas
- ❑ To perform routine screening and for diagnosing disorders of reproductive system
- ❑ To do cytohormonal study and to know the progesterone status
- ❑ To do routine examination

METHODS OF OBTAINING PAP SMEAR

- ❑ Slide method
- ❑ Liquid method

ARTICLES REQUIRED AND THEIR PURPOSES

Articles	Purposes
❑ A glass slide	
❑ A sterile spatula	❑ To separate the area
❑ Cusco's speculum	❑ To visualize
❑ A pipette	
❑ A sterile cotton swab	
❑ Sterile gloves	❑ To prevent cross infection
❑ Ether 95% alcohol solution (1:1)	❑ To clean the area
❑ Spray fixative	
❑ A graphite pencil	
❑ Light source	❑ To visualize the area
❑ K-Y jelly	❑ For smoothening

STEPS OF PROCEDURE AND RATIONALE

Steps	Rationale
❑ Check the physicians order and progress notes	❑ Obtain specific instruction/information
❑ Identify the patient against the physician's order	❑ Right procedure is performed on the right patient
❑ Explain the procedure to the patient	❑ To obtain the patient's concern and cooperation
❑ For patient of child bearing age test should be done 10–20 days after the first day of LMP and should not be done when the patient is not menstruating	❑ A smear taken other than mid menstrual cycle can result in abnormal findings
❑ Instruct the patient not to douche for 2–3 days before the test	❑ Douching may remove the exfoliated cells

Contd…

Steps	Rationale
❑ Instruct the patient not to use vaginal contraceptives or medication before 48 hours of examination. Avoid intercourse in the night before examination.	❑ Use of contraceptive before examination may lead to false result
❑ Instruct the patient to empty the bladder and rectum before the examination	❑ To ensure comfort during the procedure
Ask the patient to give following information: ❑ Age ❑ Use of contraceptive devices, birth control pills ❑ Past vaginal surgical repair or hysterectomy ❑ Any radiation therapy ❑ Any other pertinent clinical history (e.g. abnormal Pap smear signs of inflammation and bleeding)	❑ To identify patient whether the patient is an adolescent, pregnant or postmenopausal woman ❑ Hormones and other contraceptive devices can alter the findings ❑ Some medication alters the test result
Ask the patient to undress from the waist down	
Position the patient in a lithotomy position on an examination table and drape her properly	❑ To ensure good visibility and promotes comfort and provide privacy
Wear the sterile gloves lubricate and insert a cusco's speculum	
❑ For Endocervical smear (Fig. 1): Insert a sterile cotton swab into the cervical os and rotate it 360°. Leave the swab for 10–20 sec. Remove the swab and put it on to a glass slide. Fix it immediately **FIG. 1:** Endocervical smear test	
❑ Ectocervical scraping Insert Ayre's spatula into the cervical os rotate or scrape the entire surface at the squamocolumnar junction	
❑ Cervical scraping (Fig. 2) Insert the pointed edge of the wooden Ayre's spatula into the cervical os and rotate the spatula 360°. Spread the cervical scraping on a glass slide, fix it with an ether 95% ethyl alcohol solutions and dry the slide	

Contd…

Steps	Rationale
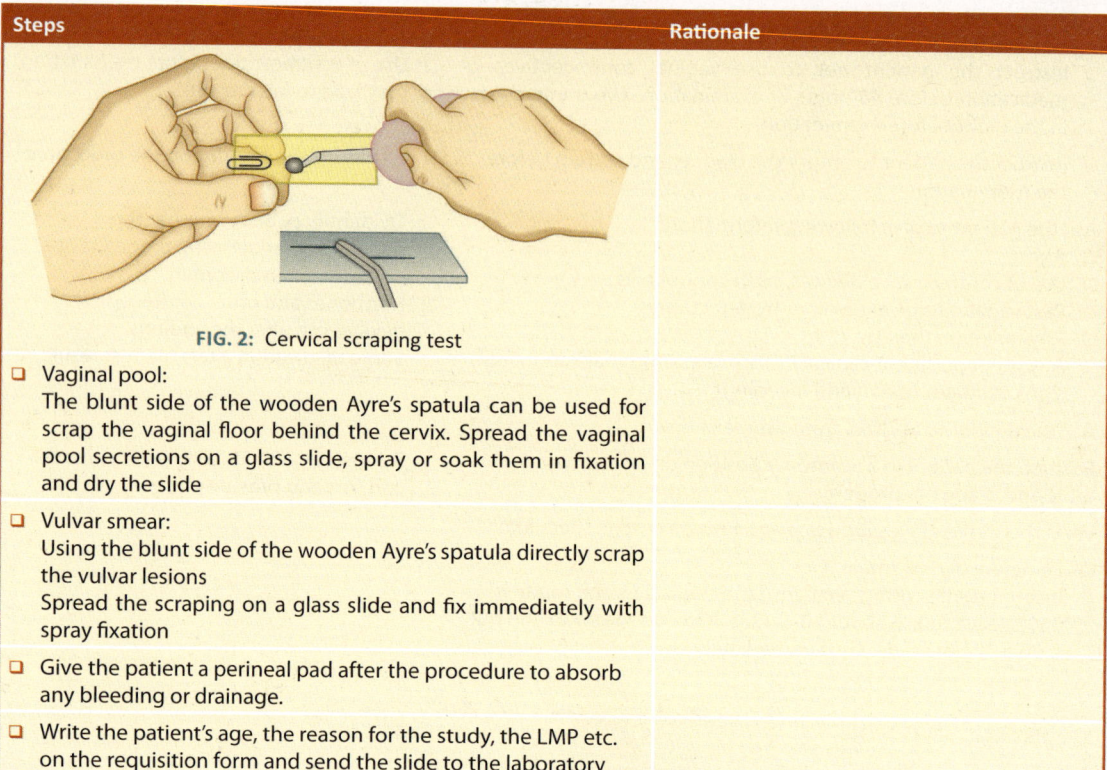 **FIG. 2:** Cervical scraping test	
❑ Vaginal pool: The blunt side of the wooden Ayre's spatula can be used for scrap the vaginal floor behind the cervix. Spread the vaginal pool secretions on a glass slide, spray or soak them in fixation and dry the slide	
❑ Vulvar smear: Using the blunt side of the wooden Ayre's spatula directly scrap the vulvar lesions Spread the scraping on a glass slide and fix immediately with spray fixation	
❑ Give the patient a perineal pad after the procedure to absorb any bleeding or drainage.	
❑ Write the patient's age, the reason for the study, the LMP etc. on the requisition form and send the slide to the laboratory	

COMPLICATIONS

❑ Infection
❑ Vaginal discharge

Points to Remember

❑ A woman may experience a small amount of spotting immediately after Pap smear.
❑ Do not lubricate the speculum as it may distort cells.

CHAPTER 25

Assisting with Lumbar Puncture

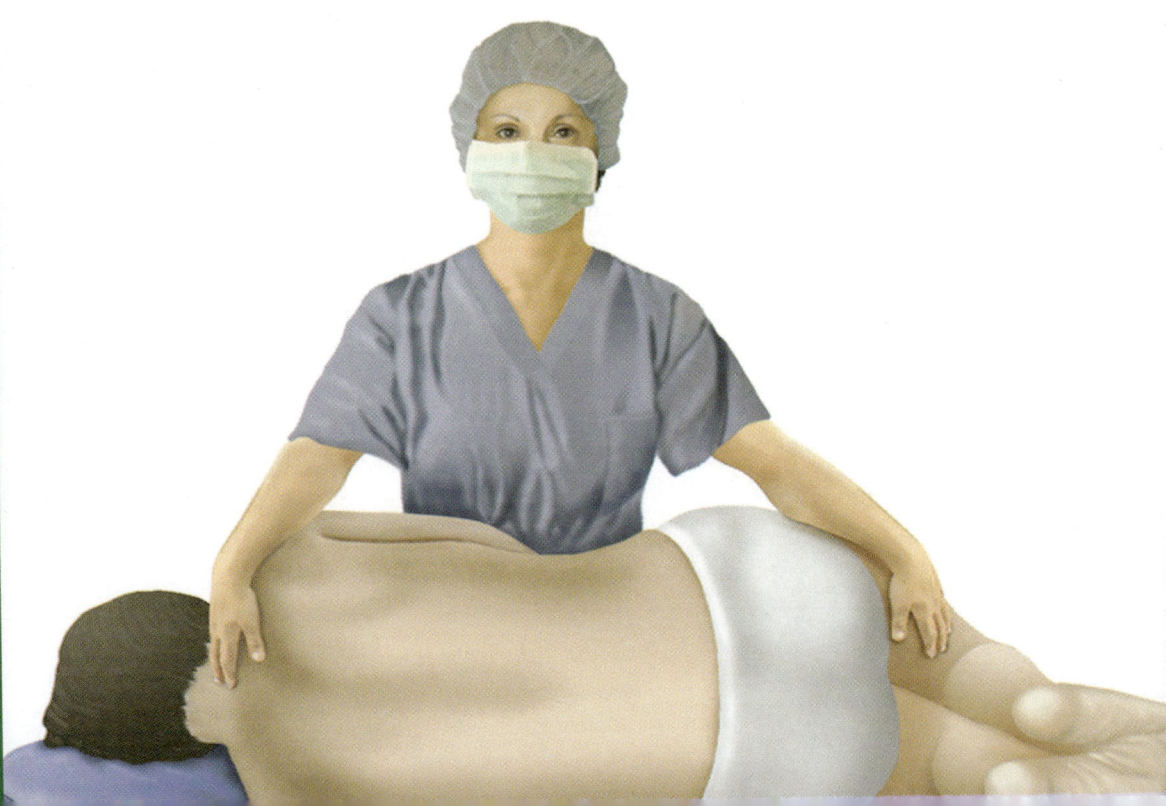

DEFINITION

Lumbar puncture is the insertion of a needle into the lumbar subarachnoid space to withdraw cerebrospinal fluid for diagnostic purpose.

PURPOSES

- ❑ To administer spinal anesthesia before surgery
- ❑ To administer medication into spinal canal of meningitis
- ❑ To reduce intracranial pressure
- ❑ To perform diagnostic studies and certain investigations
- ❑ To detect subarachnoid block

CONTRAINDICATIONS

- ❑ Suspected epidural infection
- ❑ Severe psychiatric and neuritic problems
- ❑ Chronic backache problem
- ❑ Intracranial bleeding

ARTICLES REQUIRED AND THEIR PURPOSES

Articles	Purposes
A sterile tray containing (LP set):	
❑ LP needle with stillette	❑ To puncture the site
❑ Sponge holding forceps	❑ To hold the needle
❑ Small bowls	❑ To keep the cotton
❑ Specimens bottles	❑ To collect the fluid
❑ Cotton balls, gauze pieces, cotton pads	❑ To clean the area
❑ Dressing articles	❑ To do the dressing after the procedure
❑ A clean tray containing: Macintosh and towel	❑ To prevent from soiling of the bed
❑ Kidney tray/paper bag	❑ To collect the waste
❑ Spirit iodine, tincture benzoin	❑ To clean the site
❑ Lignocaine 2%	❑ To provide local anesthesia
❑ Sterile normal saline	
❑ Adhesive plaster and scissors	
❑ Sterile gloves, gown and mask	
❑ 3-way adapter manometer and tubing	❑ To stop the CSF leakage
❑ Syringe and needle	❑ For local anesthesia

STEPS OF PROCEDURE AND RATIONALE

Steps	Rationale
❑ Explain the procedure to the patient	❑ To allay anxiety and fear of the patient
❑ Instruct the patient to void before the procedure	❑ To make patient comfortable
❑ Instruct the patient not to make any movements during the procedure	❑ To avoid injury to the spinal cord and its nerves
❑ Check the vitals of the patient	❑ It helps in obtaining baseline data
❑ Position the patient on one side at the edge of the bed with back toward the physician. Make the patient to lie down in the C-Shaped position (Fig. 1). The head and neck are flexed and brought toward chest. Keep both hands between the knees	❑ Flexion of the thighs and legs increases the space between vertebrae and facilitates easy entry of needle into the subarachnoid space

FIG. 1: C-shaped position of the patient

FIG. 2: Pillow under the head of patient to maintain the spine under horizontal position

Steps	Rationale
❑ Keep a pillow under the head (Fig. 2)	❑ It maintains the spine under horizontal position
❑ Encourage the patient to be relax and take long breath during the procedure. Do not allow the patient to talk	❑ Hyperventilation may cause an error in pressure reading
❑ Fold back the upper garments above the waist line and lower garments below the hip for exposing the site	❑ Avoid over exposure of the patient
❑ Assist the physician in cleaning the puncture site with antiseptic solution and injecting local anesthesia	❑ Prevent risk of getting infection
❑ Spinal needle is inserted into the subarachnoid space by physician through the 3rd, 4th and 5th lumbar intercostal space	
❑ Physician removes stylet and connects three-way stop cock with manometer filled with normal saline	❑ Normal pressure is 6–13 mm of mercury or 80–180 cm of water

Contd…

Assisting with Lumbar Puncture

Steps	Rationale
❑ Collect the CSF specimen into 3 specimen bottles after measuring pressure	
❑ Needle is withdrawn by the physician	
❑ Assist the physician in sealing the puncture site with tincture benzoin and apply sterile dressing	❑ Dressing protects and prevents the leakage of CSF fluid from the puncture site
❑ Instruct the patient to be flat for 12–24 hours	❑ It helps to decrease the CSF pressure in the caudal area where the needle insertion is occurred and decreases the risk of leakage
❑ Monitor the complications of lumbar puncture, check the vital signs every half an hour for 3–4 hours till stable	❑ Postlumbar headache may appear a few hours to several days after the procedure
❑ Check puncture site for CSF leakage	
❑ Encourage the patient to take more fluids after the procedure	❑ Reduces the risk of postlumbar headache
❑ Record the procedure with date, time, CSF, pressure amount drawn color nature of CSF, and general condition of patient during and after the procedure	
❑ Send the specimen to the laboratory with proper labels and requisition forms	❑ Detects chemical, bacteriological and cellular composition of CSF and helps to diagnose the disease
❑ If no complications observed give upright position to the patient after 24 hours	

COMPLICATIONS

❑ CSF leakage
❑ Infection
❑ Postpuncture headache
❑ Paralysis
❑ Hematoma

Points to Remember

❑ See that there should not be the CSF leakage.
❑ Check for any post puncture headache.
❑ Assess for paralysis attack.

Principles and Procedures of NURSING FOUNDATIONS

CHAPTER 26

Assisting Patient with Continuous Ambulatory Peritoneal Dialysis

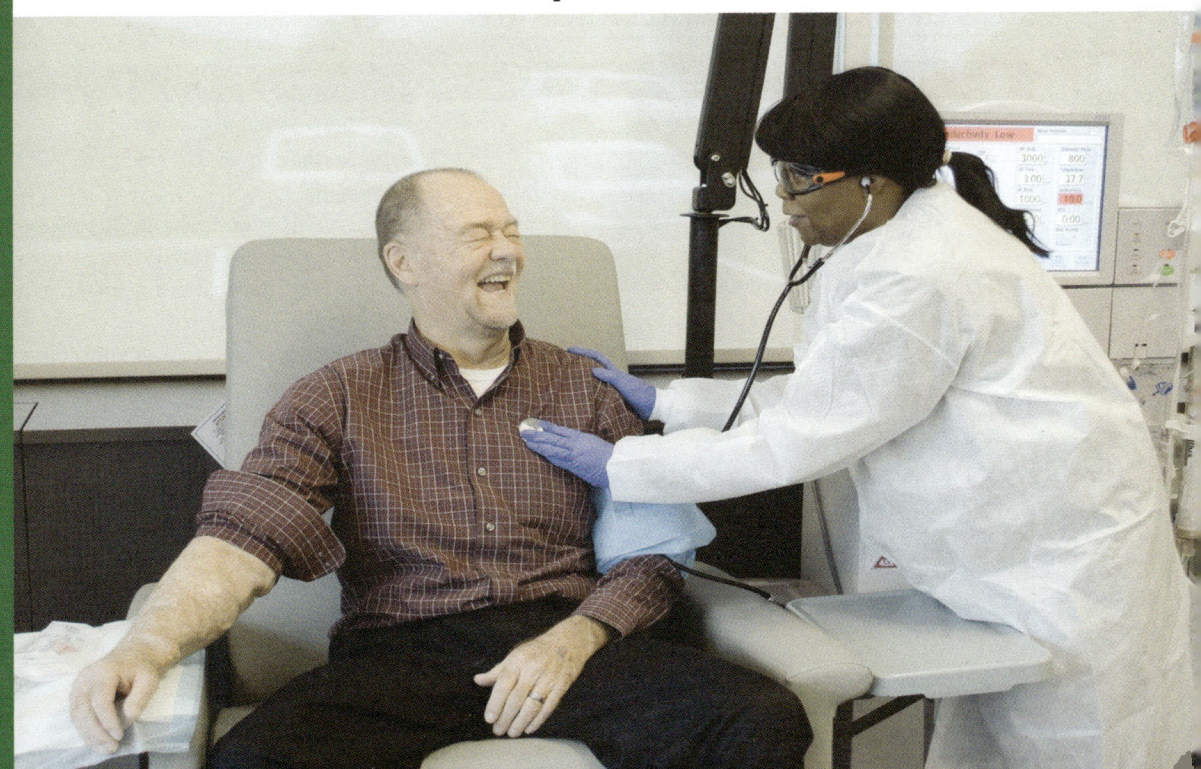

DEFINITION

Continuous peritoneal dialysis is a procedure in which peritoneal catheter is implanted through the abdominal tunnel to provide protection against bacterial infection, dialyzate, flow on the principle of gravity.

PURPOSES

- To maintain fluid balance
- To maintain adequate nutrition
- To reduce nitrogenous waste
- To maintain electrolyte and acid-base balance
- To prevent infection
- To achieve an acceptable quality of life within the constraints of a lifelong state of chronic illness.

ARTICLES REQUIRED AND THEIR PURPOSES

Articles	Purposes
Dialysis administration set or kit	To perform peritoneal dialysis
Peritoneal dialysis solution supplementary drugs as required	To separate the waste product from the peritoneal fluid
Local anesthesia	To reduce pain
CVP monitoring equipment	To maintain normal CVP pressure
Suture set	To suture the site after procedure
Sterile gloves	To reduce cross infection
Antiseptic solution	To reduce infection

STEPS OF PROCEDURE AND RATIONALE

Steps	Rationale
Explain the procedure to the patient	To gain confidence and cooperation
Check the vital signs of the patient	To compare the subsequent changes
Make sure the patient is on empty bladder	If the bladder is empty there is less chances of perforating when the trocar is introduced into the peritoneum
Flush the tubing with dialysis solution	The tubing is flushed to prevent air from entering peritoneal cavity
Provide comfortable supine position to the patient	This protect the patient from air born contamination
The abdomen is prepared surgically and the skin and subcutaneous tissues are infiltrated with local anesthesia	To reduce pain during insertion of trocar in the abdomen
A small midline stab wound is made 3–5 cm below the umbilicus. The trocar is inserted through the incision	It helps accurately to know where to insert the trocar
The patient is requested to raise his head from the pillow after the trocar is introduced	This helps to tighten the abdominal muscles and permits easier penetration of the trocar

Contd…

Steps	Rationale
❑ Dialysis fluid is allowed to run through the catheter while it is being positioned (Fig. 1) 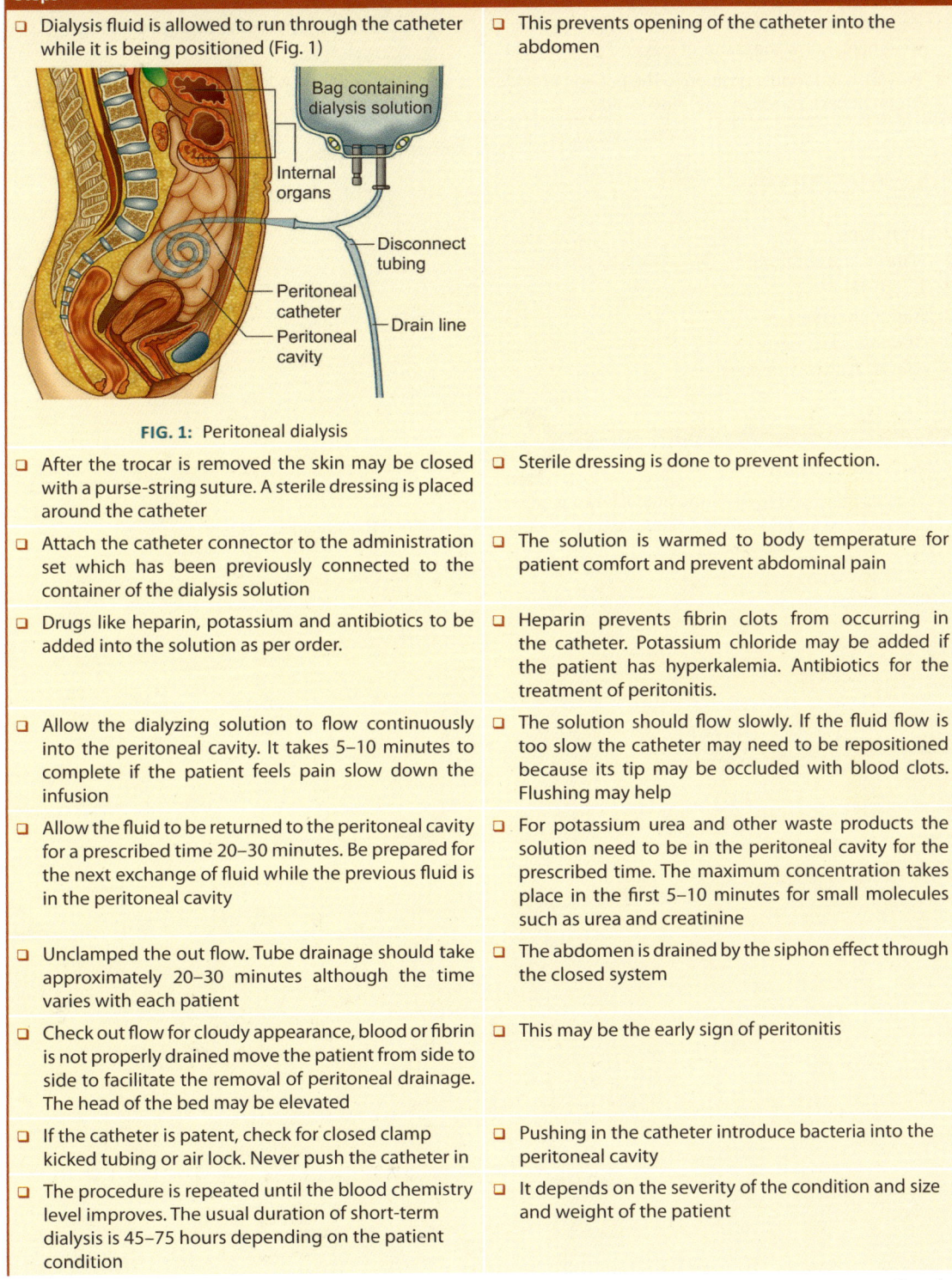 FIG. 1: Peritoneal dialysis	❑ This prevents opening of the catheter into the abdomen
❑ After the trocar is removed the skin may be closed with a purse-string suture. A sterile dressing is placed around the catheter	❑ Sterile dressing is done to prevent infection.
❑ Attach the catheter connector to the administration set which has been previously connected to the container of the dialysis solution	❑ The solution is warmed to body temperature for patient comfort and prevent abdominal pain
❑ Drugs like heparin, potassium and antibiotics to be added into the solution as per order.	❑ Heparin prevents fibrin clots from occurring in the catheter. Potassium chloride may be added if the patient has hyperkalemia. Antibiotics for the treatment of peritonitis.
❑ Allow the dialyzing solution to flow continuously into the peritoneal cavity. It takes 5–10 minutes to complete if the patient feels pain slow down the infusion	❑ The solution should flow slowly. If the fluid flow is too slow the catheter may need to be repositioned because its tip may be occluded with blood clots. Flushing may help
❑ Allow the fluid to be returned to the peritoneal cavity for a prescribed time 20–30 minutes. Be prepared for the next exchange of fluid while the previous fluid is in the peritoneal cavity	❑ For potassium urea and other waste products the solution need to be in the peritoneal cavity for the prescribed time. The maximum concentration takes place in the first 5–10 minutes for small molecules such as urea and creatinine
❑ Unclamped the out flow. Tube drainage should take approximately 20–30 minutes although the time varies with each patient	❑ The abdomen is drained by the siphon effect through the closed system
❑ Check out flow for cloudy appearance, blood or fibrin is not properly drained move the patient from side to side to facilitate the removal of peritoneal drainage. The head of the bed may be elevated	❑ This may be the early sign of peritonitis
❑ If the catheter is patent, check for closed clamp kicked tubing or air lock. Never push the catheter in	❑ Pushing in the catheter introduce bacteria into the peritoneal cavity
❑ The procedure is repeated until the blood chemistry level improves. The usual duration of short-term dialysis is 45–75 hours depending on the patient condition	❑ It depends on the severity of the condition and size and weight of the patient

Contd…

Assisting Patient with Continuous Ambulatory Peritoneal Dialysis

Steps	Rationale
❑ Keep the exact record of patient fluid balance during treatment. Know the status of loss and gain of fluid	❑ Complications may occur with large fluid loss
❑ Provide comfortable position to the patient. Provide frequent back care turn from side to side	❑ The dialysis period is lengthy and the patient becomes fatigued

COMPLICATIONS

❑ Peritonitis
❑ Nausea and vomiting
❑ Anorexia
❑ Abdominal pain
❑ Abdominal tenderness
❑ Cloudy dialysis drainage

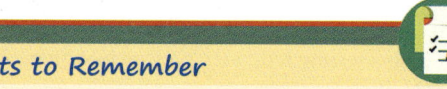

Points to Remember

❑ Dialysis may need to be terminated if leakage persist.
❑ Observe the abdominal pain, note the time of discomfort and seal the leakage.

CHAPTER 27

Assisting with Insertion of Sengstaken-Blakemore Tube Balloon Tamponade

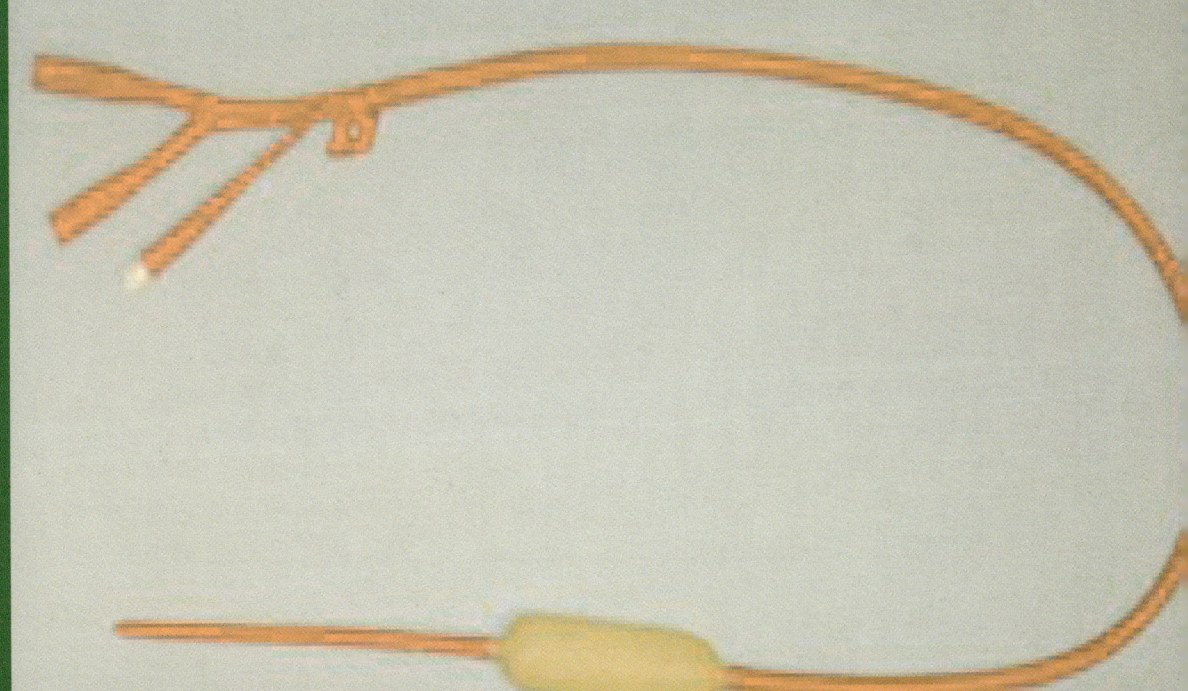

DEFINITION

Assisting in insertion of Sengstaken-Blakemore tube which exerts pressure directly on bleeding sites and stomach.

TYPES OF TUBES USD FOR TAMPONADE AND THEIR PARTS

- ❑ Sengstaken-blakemore tube
  - ○ Esophageal balloon
  - ○ Gastric balloon
  - ○ Gastric aspiration port
- ❑ Minnesota tube
  - ○ Esophageal tube
  - ○ Gastric balloon
  - ○ Gastric aspiration port
  - ○ Esophageal aspiration port

PURPOSE

- ❑ To arrest acute bleeding from esophageal varices and stomach.

ARTICLES REQUIRED AND THEIR PURPOSES

Articles	Purposes
❑ Sengstaken-Blakemore tube (Fig. 1)	❑ To insert the tube into the esophagus

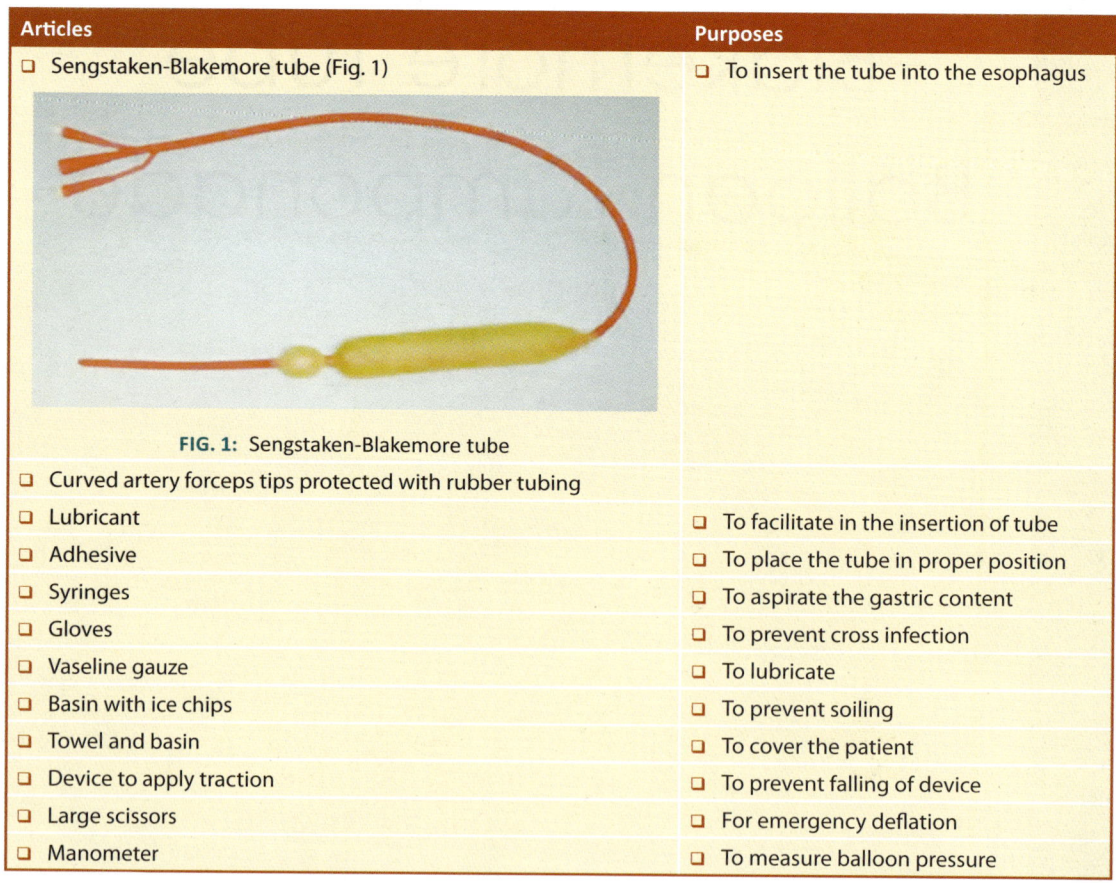

FIG. 1: Sengstaken-Blakemore tube

Articles	Purposes
❑ Curved artery forceps tips protected with rubber tubing	
❑ Lubricant	❑ To facilitate in the insertion of tube
❑ Adhesive	❑ To place the tube in proper position
❑ Syringes	❑ To aspirate the gastric content
❑ Gloves	❑ To prevent cross infection
❑ Vaseline gauze	❑ To lubricate
❑ Basin with ice chips	❑ To prevent soiling
❑ Towel and basin	❑ To cover the patient
❑ Device to apply traction	❑ To prevent falling of device
❑ Large scissors	❑ For emergency deflation
❑ Manometer	❑ To measure balloon pressure

STEPS OF PROCEDURE AND RATIONALE

Steps	Rationale
❑ Explain the procedure to the patient and give psychological support	❑ It helps in obtaining cooperation from the patient
❑ Elevate head end of the bed slightly unless the patient is in shock	
❑ Check balloon by trail inflation to detect leaks	❑ This is best done because it is easier to see escaping of air bubbles
❑ Lubricate the tube before the physician passes it via mouth or nose	❑ Lubrication lessens friction of the tube
❑ Allow the patient to drink few sips of water	❑ It will help in making the passage of the tube
❑ Placement of the tube in the stomach can be verified by irrigating the gastric tube with air while auscultating over the stomach	❑ It indicates that the tube is in stomach so that the gastric tube is not inflated in the esophagus
❑ An X-ray of lower chest and upper abdomen can be obtained to verify placement of the tube in the stomach. Then inflate gastric balloon with air and gently pull tube back to seat balloon against gastroesophageal junction	❑ It helps to exert pressure on cardiac sphincter
❑ Clamp gastric balloon tube and mark tube location at nares	❑ Prevents air leakage from the tube and mark allows easy visualization of movement of the tube.
❑ Apply gentle traction to the balloon and secure it with a foam rubber cube at the nares	❑ It prevents the tube from displacement and assists in exerting adequate pressure
❑ A 'Y' connector is attached to esophageal balloon opening. Attach syringe to one arm of the 'y' connector and manometer to the other. Inflate esophageal balloon to 25–35 mm Hg pressure (Fig. 2)	

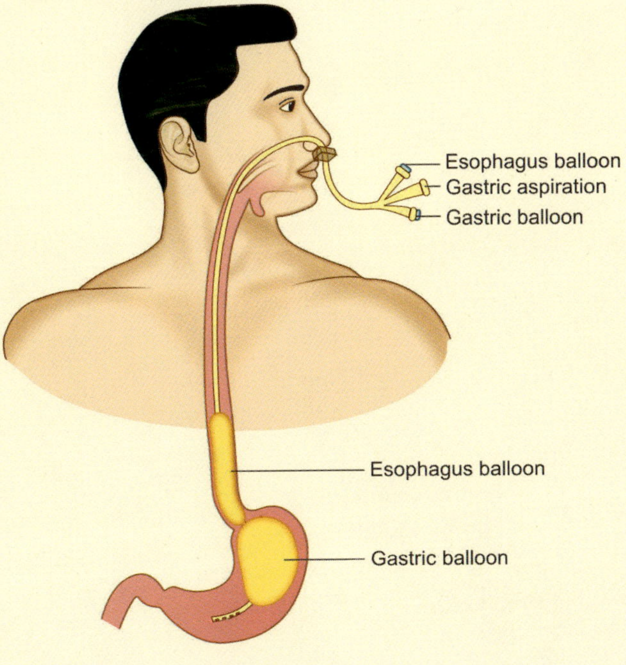

Esophagus balloon
Gastric aspiration
Gastric balloon

Esophagus balloon

Gastric balloon

FIG. 2: 'Y' connector attached to esophageal balloon

Contd…

Assisting with Insertion of Sengstaken-Blakemore Tube Balloon Tamponade

Steps	Rationale
❑ Suctioning is done to aspirate the gastric content for every hourly	❑ It helps to remove old blood from the stomach and prevent hepatic encephalopathy
❑ Insert a nasogastric tube positioning it above the esophageal balloon and attach to suction	❑ It serves to check for bleeding and suctions saliva accumulated above the esophageal balloon
❑ Label each port ❑ Tape a scissors at head of bed	❑ To prevent accidental or irrigation airway. Occlusion may occur if the esophageal balloon is pulled into the hypopharynx. If this occurs the esophageal balloon tube must be cut and removed immediately

Points to Remember

- ❑ Maintain constant vigilance while balloons are inflated in the patient.
- ❑ Keep balloon pressures at required level to control bleeding.
- ❑ Observe and record vital signs, monitor color and amount of NG lavage fluid for evidence of bleeding.

CHAPTER 28

Colostomy Care

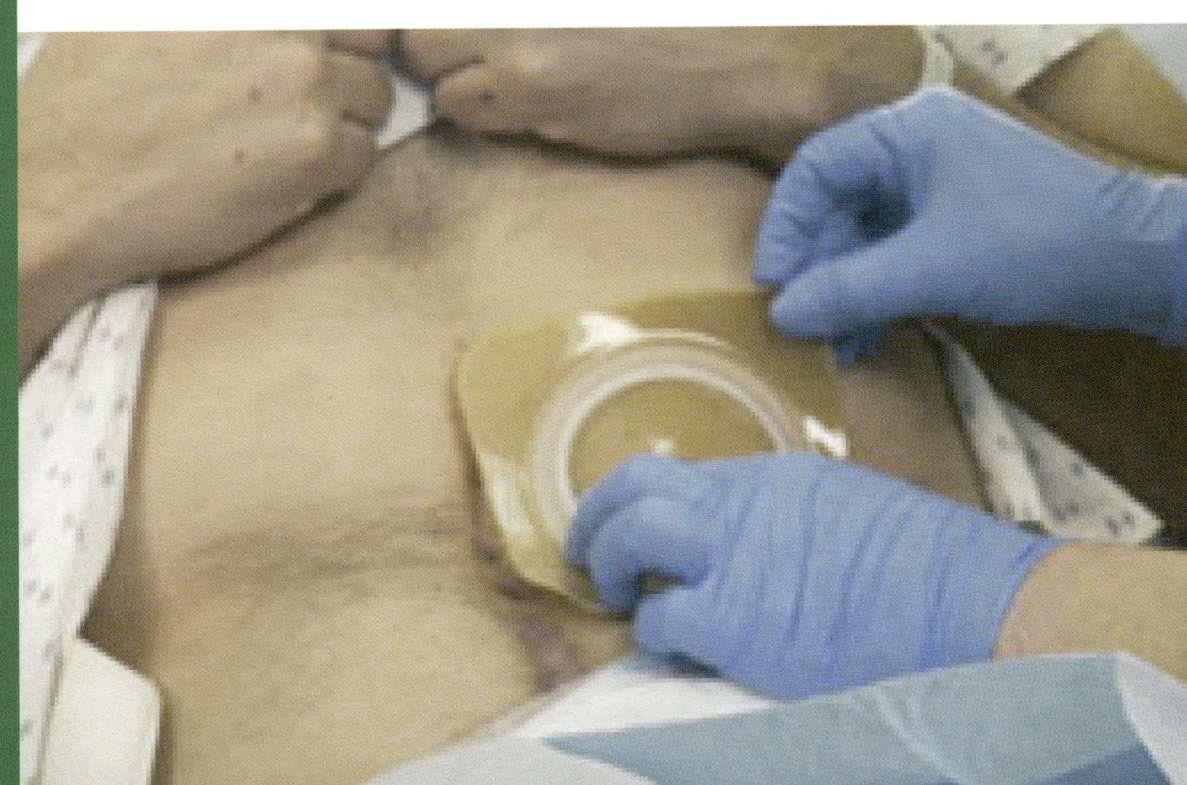

DEFINITION

An ostomy is a surgically created opening between intestines and abdominal wall.

Ostomy is performed when bowel and bladder dysfunction occurs due to disease conditions, injury or congenital deformity.

INDICATIONS

- Colorectal cancer
- Bladder cancer
- Crohn's disease
- Ulcerative colitis
- Congenital defects
- Other intestinal/urinary conditions
- Removal of bladder

TYPES

Three types of ostomies are as follows:
- **Colostomy:** Connects a part of large intestine to the abdominal wall.
- **Ileostomy:** Connects the last part of small intestine (ileum) to the abdominal wall.
- **Urostomy:** Connects the one or both ureters from kidney to the abdominal wall.

PURPOSES

- To prevent leakage
- To prevent excoriation of skin and stoma
- To observe stoma and surrounding skin
- To teach patient and relatives about stoma care and collection bag

ARTICLES REQUIRED AND THEIR PURPOSES

Articles	Purposes
A clean tray containing:	
Disposable colostomy bag	To change the colostomy bag
Mackintosh with draw sheet	To prevent soiling of linen
Pair of clean gloves	To prevent cross infection
Normal saline/basin with warm tap water	To rinse the colostomy pouch
Gauze pieces	
Skin barrier cream	To protect skin from irritation
Kidney tray/paper bag	To collect waste materials
Stoma measuring guide	Ensures accurate size of pouch
Scissor and pen	
Bed pan with lid	To collect fecal matter

PRELIMINARY ASSESSMENT

Preparation of the Patient

☐ Identify the patient and explain the procedure to gain cooperation.
☐ Assess the skin integrity around the stoma.
☐ Note the amount and character of fecal material in the stoma pouch.

STEPS OF PROCEDURE AND RATIONALE

Steps	Rationale
☐ Arrange all the articles at the bedside	☐ To save energy and time
☐ Provide privacy	☐ To make patient comfortable
☐ Give comfortable position to the patient	☐ For smooth performance of procedure
☐ Wash hands and wear gloves	☐ To prevent infection
☐ Spread Mackintosh and draw sheet	☐ To protect linen
☐ Remove used pouch and skin barrier gently by pushing the skin away from the barrier	☐ Reduces trauma and irritation to the skin
☐ Empty the contents into the bed pan, if it is drainable	☐ To accidental spillage of fecal matter
☐ Slowly remove the appliance from the stoma if any resistance is felt use warm water to facilitate removal	☐ Minimize discomfort to the patient
☐ Clean the excess stool from stoma gauze piece and cover the stoma with fresh piece of gauze. (If needed we can gently wash the stoma surrounding by mild cleansing agents as per hospital protocol)	
☐ Do not scrub the skin, dry completely by patting the skin with gauze and cover stoma with gauze	☐ Stoma surface is highly vascular. Skin barrier does not adhere to wet skin.
☐ Observe stoma for color, swelling, trauma and healing. Stoma should be moist and pink	☐ To find out complications such as altered circulation
☐ Measure the stoma using measuring guide to select the size	☐ Ensures accuracy of pouch size
☐ Trace same size circle behind the skin barrier, using scissors, cut an opening 1/4–1/8 inch larger than stoma	
☐ Put skin barrier and pouch over the stoma, and gently press on to the skin. Hold the pouch in place for 3–5 minutes.	☐ Easy application of pouch
☐ As per hospital protocol, use deodorant in bag if required	
☐ Remove gloves and wash hands	☐ Prevent cross infection
☐ Make the patient comfortable	
☐ Clean the area and replace all articles ☐ Record the procedure with following details: Appearance of stoma, peristomal skin, amount, color, and consistency of the fecal matter in the pouch.	☐ Helps in continuation of care
Emptying bag without changing: ☐ Empty fecal matter into the bedpan ☐ Rinse the pouch with warm water as much as required ☐ Spray deodorant into pouch. Uncuff the pouch and apply the clamp ☐ Discard the waste materials in appropriate bin ☐ Remove gloves and wash hands ☐ Record the observation, procedure and patients response	 ☐ Minimize odor ☐ Clean appearance ☐ Prevent bad odor. Clamp secures appliance. ☐ Prevent spread of microorganisms ☐ Helps in continuation of care

Colostomy Care

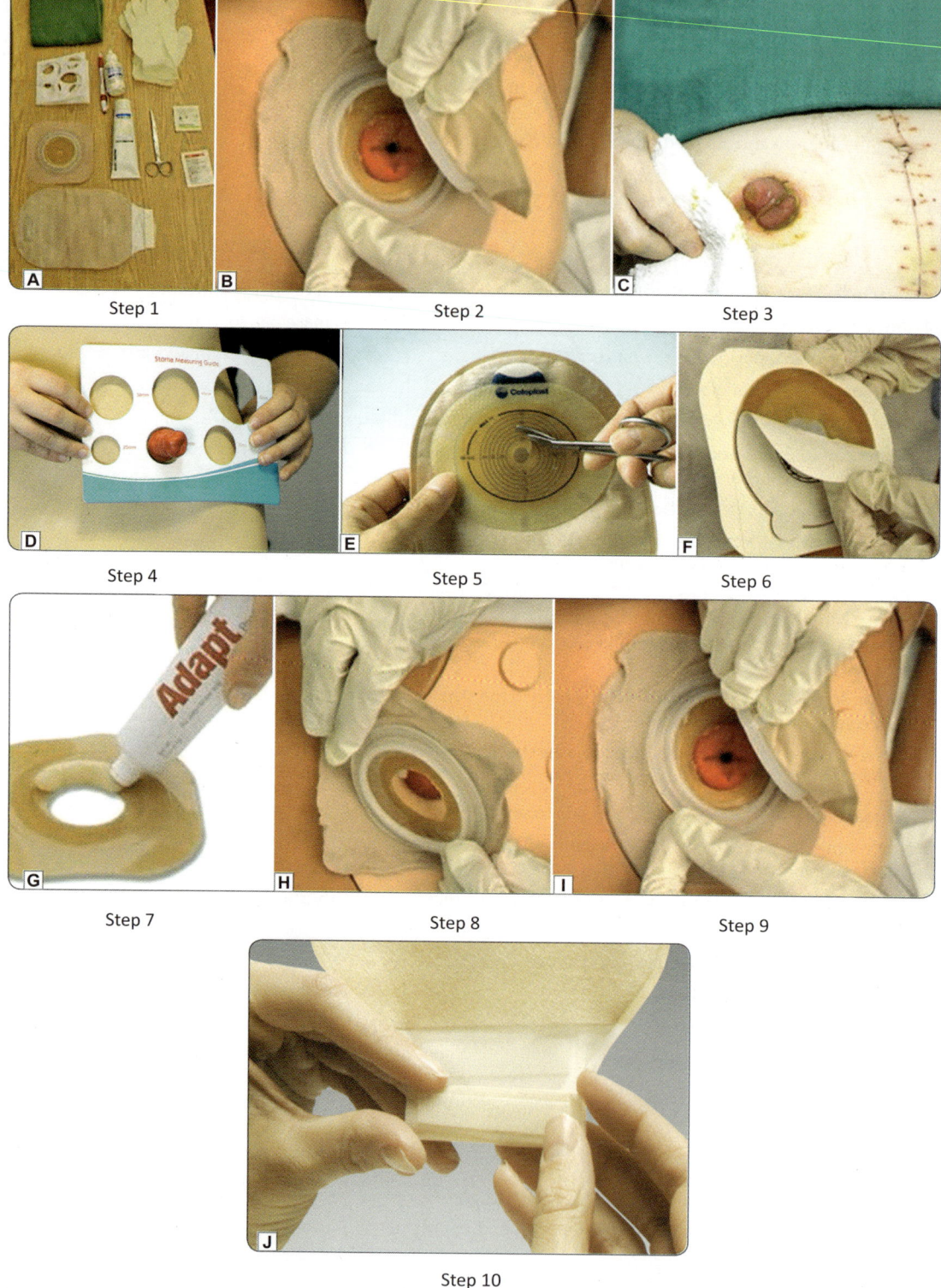

Step 1 Step 2 Step 3

Step 4 Step 5 Step 6

Step 7 Step 8 Step 9

Step 10

FIGS 1A TO J: 10 steps of changing a colostomy bag

Points to Remember

- Monitor intake output strictly.
- Check stoma appliance for quantity and quality of discharge.
- Keep stoma site dry always as moisture increases chance for infection.
- Advice patient to avoid gas containing food in their diet.

NOTES

CHAPTER 29

Intracranial Pressure Monitoring

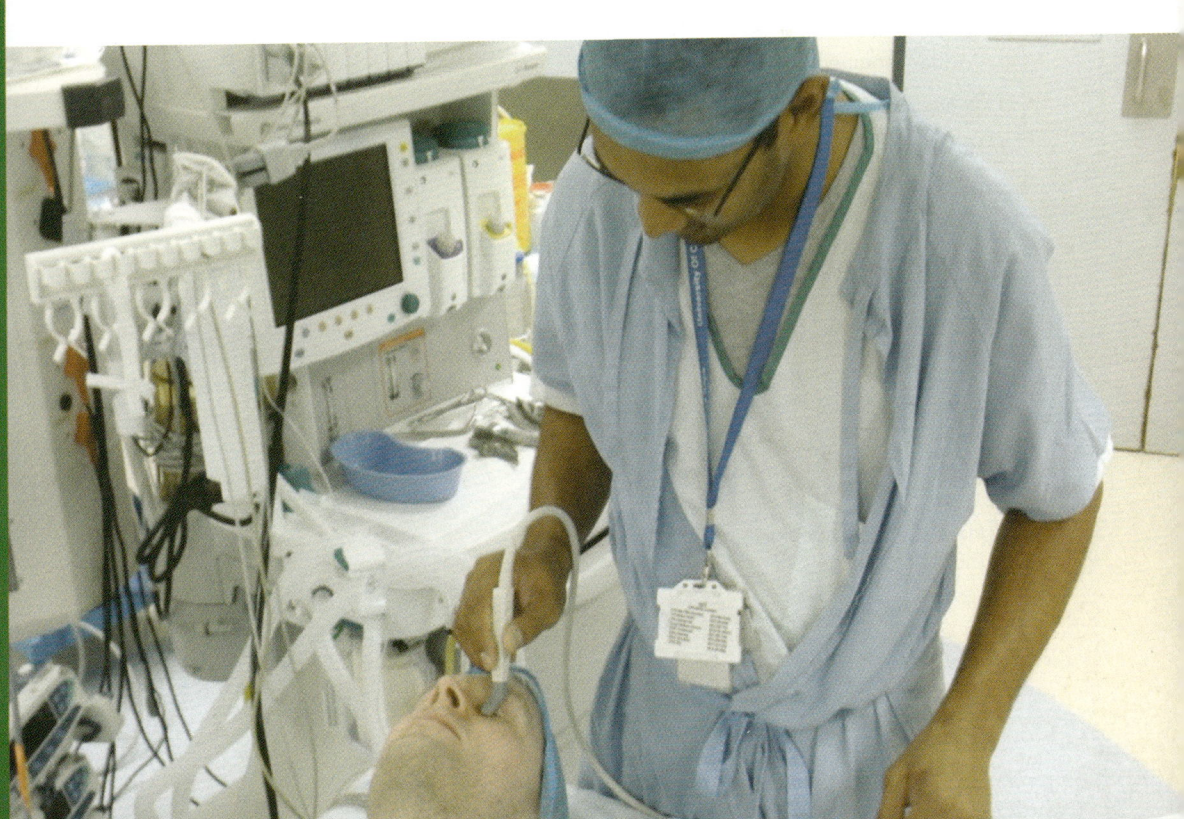

DEFINITION

Intracranial pressure (ICP) monitoring measures the pressure exerted by the brain blood and CSF fluid against the inner wall of the skull.

PURPOSES

- ❑ Head trauma with bleeding or edema
- ❑ Overproduction or insufficient absorption of CSF
- ❑ Cerebral hemorrhage and space occupying lesion.

CLASSIFICATION

- ❑ Intraventricular catheter monitoring
- ❑ Subarachnoid blood monitoring
- ❑ Epidural or subdural sensor monitoring
- ❑ Intraparenchymal monitoring

ARTICLES REQUIRED AND THEIR PURPOSES

Articles	Purposes
❑ Monitoring unit and transducers as ordered	❑ To measure the ICP with the device
❑ Sterile gauze 4 × 4 inches 16–20	❑ To cover the site
❑ Mackintosh	❑ To prevent soiling of the linen
❑ Shaving kit	❑ To remove hairs of the skull
❑ Sterile drapes	❑ To cover the head
❑ Povidone iodine solutions	❑ To prevent from infection
❑ Two pairs of sterile gloves	❑ To avoid cross infection
❑ Head dressing supplies (2 rolls of 4" elastic gauze dressing, 1 roll of 4 roller gauze adhesive tape)	❑ To cover the wound

STEPS OF PROCEDURE AND RATIONALE

Steps	Rationale
❑ Provide privacy to the patient if the procedure is being done in the open emergency department or intensive care unit	❑ To avoid unwanted exposure of the patient to other unit members
❑ Obtain baseline routine and neurological vital signs	❑ To aid in prompt detection of disease during the procedure
❑ Place the client in the supine position and elevate the head of the bed at 30°	❑ It helps in proper monitoring

Contd…

Steps	Rationale
❑ Place Mackintosh under the patient head. Shave or clip his hair at the insertion site as indicated by the doctor to decrease the risk of infection (Figs 1 and 2) 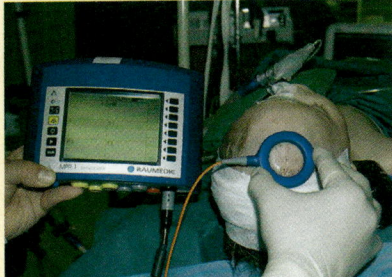 **FIG. 1:** Shave hair at the insertion site	❑ To avoid soiling of the linen

❑ Carefully fold and remove the device, hold the client head in your hand or attach a long strip of 4" roller gauze to one side rail

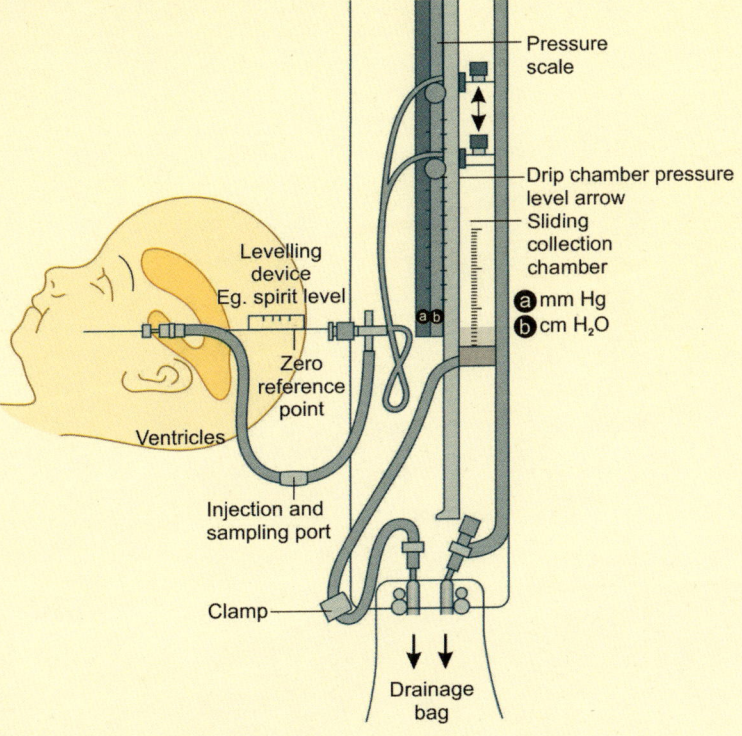

FIG. 2: Intracranial pressure monitoring

❑ Observe for cardiac arrhythmias and abnormal respiratory pattern	
❑ After insertion apply povidone iodine solution and a sterile dressing to the site it not done by the doctor	
❑ If the doctor has set up a drainage system attach the drip chamber to the head board or bedside IV pole as ordered.	

Intracranial Pressure Monitoring

AFTER CARE

- ❑ Positioning the drip chamber too high may raise ICP. Positioning it too low may cause excessive CSF drainage
- ❑ Inspect the insertion site at least every 24 hours for redness swelling and drainage
- ❑ Calculate cerebral perfusion pressure (CPP) hourly use the equation

$$CPP = MAP - ICP$$

MAP refers to mean arterial pressure.

Point to Remember

- ❑ Clean the site repeatedly with povidone iodine solution and apply a fresh sterile dressing.

CHAPTER 30

Cerebrospinal Fluid Flow Monitoring

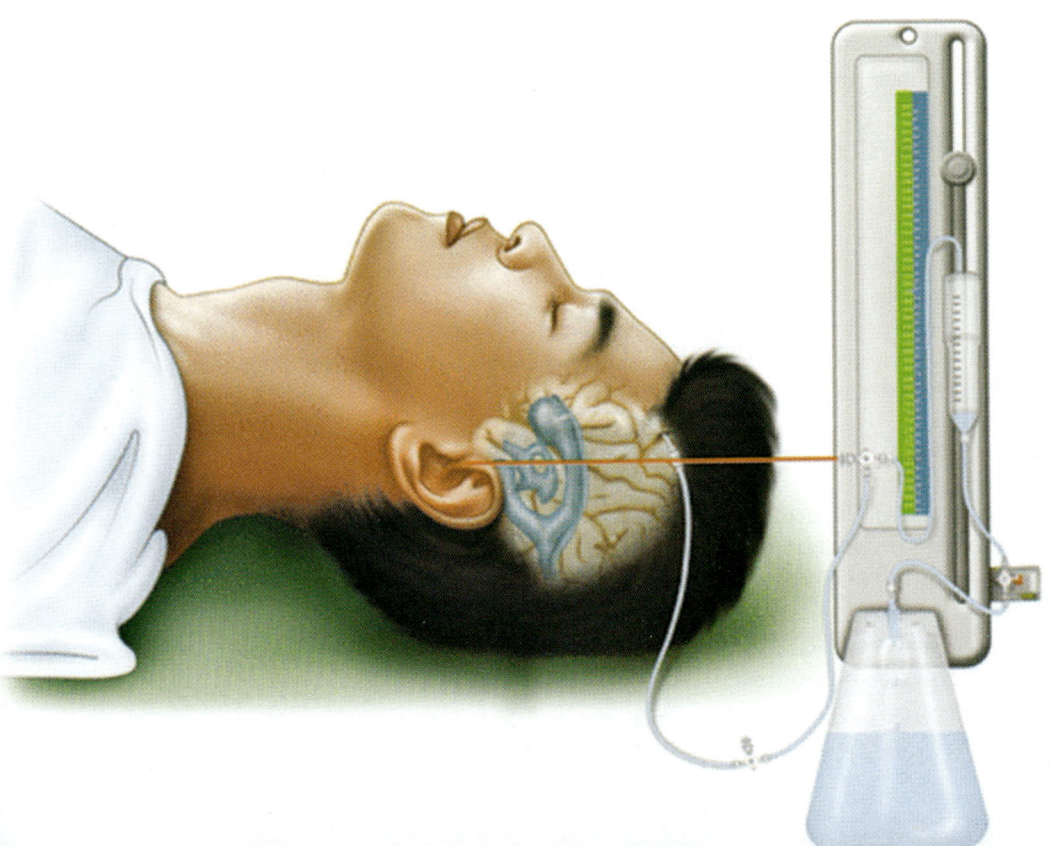

INTRODUCTION

Cerebrospinal fluid (CSF) flow monitoring is a nuclear study performed to evaluate patency and filtering of the CSF Pathways and the reabsorption or leakage of CSF.

It is the most important procedure used to diagnose surgically treatable hydrocephalus and to evaluate shunt patency postoperatively.

Reference values: **Normal CSF** value : Total protein: 15 to 60 mg/100 mL. Gamma globulin: 3% to 12% of the total protein. CSF glucose: 50 to 80 mg/100 ml, CSF cell count: 0 to 5 white blood cells and no red blood cells.

Interfering factors: Inability of the client to remain still during the procedure especially if the client is a child.

INDICATIONS

❑ To diagnose and differentiate between communicating nonobstructive hydrocephalus in infants revealed by reflux into the ventricles respectively.

❑ Evaluating the size of the ventricles with CSF reflux if an obstruction is present or evaluating the ability to reabsorb the fluid revealed by an increase uptake of the radionuclide in the ventricles.

❑ Determining spinal masses lesions.

❑ Evaluating preoperatively for shunt type and placement and postoperatively for shunt patency and effectiveness.

CONTRAINDICATIONS

Pregnancy unless the benefits of performing the procedure greatly outweigh the risk to the fetus.

NURSING CARE BEFORE THE PROCEDURE

❑ Teaching should include information about the route of the radiopharmaceutical administration and explanation of the procedure.

❑ Inform the client that the schedule of delayed studies may continue up to 3 days and that no medication are administered before the procedure

❑ Maintain the client in a supine position after the lumbar puncture

NURSING CARE DURING THE PROCEDURE

❑ The client is placed flat on the examination table in a supine position 1 hour after injection of the radiopharmaceutical into the spinal column. A head down position is also provided sometimes.

❑ The client is reminded to live very still while the scanner is operating. The scanner is moved over the head for imaging of ventricular flow.

❑ Subsequent imaging takes place in 4, 6, 24, 28, and 72 hours depending on persistent reflux.

❑ Anteroposterior vertex and lateral views are made with client position changed as needed for the desired projections.

NURSING CARE AFTER THE PROCEDURE

❑ Assess the puncture site for leakage and apply a small dressing

❑ Return the client to the hospital room in a prone position

❑ Instruct the client to maintain a prone or supine position for 4–8 hours after the study.

Points to Remember

❑ Should monitor respiratory function in every 10–5 minutes.

❑ Monitor neurological status to avoid complications.

CHAPTER 31

Pacemaker Implantation Procedure

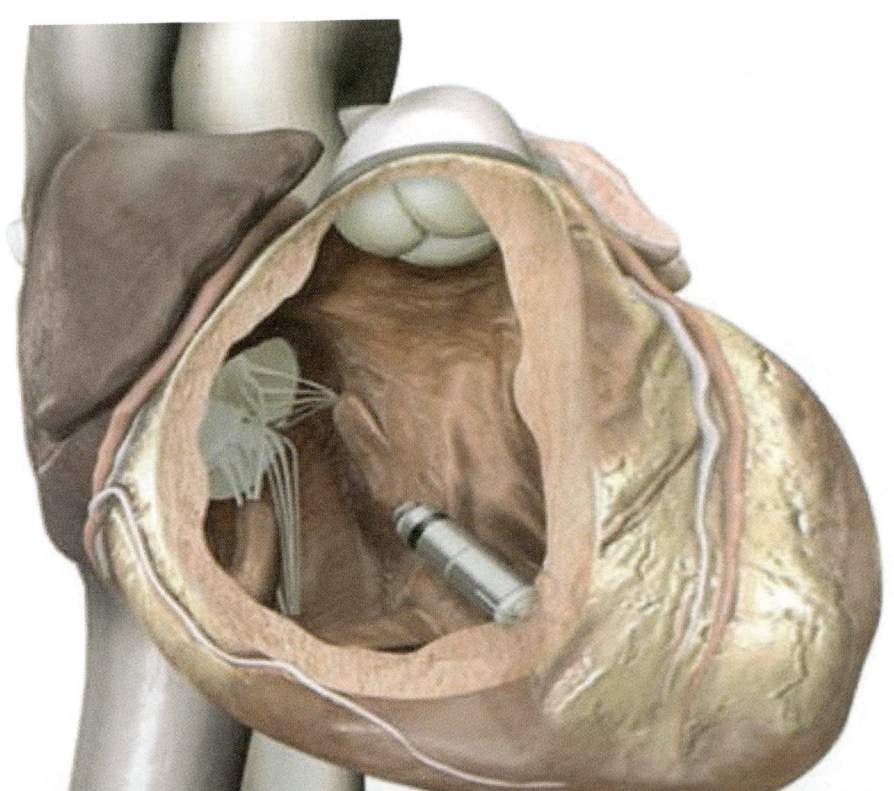

DEFINITION

An artificial pacemaker is a mechanical device that electronically stimulates electrical impulses initiation within the heart.

PURPOSES

- ❑ To treat the partial or complete heart block which does not respond to the drug therapy
- ❑ To correct abnormal drug resistant bradycardias rhythm of the heart
- ❑ To generate the electrical signals between both the ventricles
- ❑ To coordinate electrical signals between the upper and lower chambers of the heart

TYPES

- ❑ Temporary pacemaker
- ❑ Permanent pacemaker

Based on the Place of Action

- ❑ Stimulation of ventricles only required
- ❑ QRS inhibited demand pacing
- ❑ P wave triggered ventricle pacing
- ❑ Stimulation of atria required in the presence of normal conduction
- ❑ If stimulation of both atria is required

INDICATIONS

- ❑ Arrhythmias–atrial fibrillation
- ❑ Symptomatic sinus bradycardia
- ❑ Certain congenital heart disorders
- ❑ Heart failure with ejection fraction <35%
- ❑ Heart transplants
- ❑ History of cardiac arrest
- ❑ Long QT syndrome
- ❑ Syncope
- ❑ Tachycardia
- ❑ Third degree AV block with slow ventricular rate
- ❑ Right bundle branch block (RBBB)

COMPLICATIONS

- ❑ Dislodgment of lead—occurs in 2.5% of patients
- ❑ Malposition—usually occurs with patients with atrial or ventricular septal defects
- ❑ Venous thrombosis—occurs in up to 40% of patients; symptoms include neck discomfort, swelling of the arms, face, and head
- ❑ Device problems—conductor failure, insulator failure
- ❑ Abnormal heart rhythms
- ❑ Bleeding
- ❑ Punctured lung
- ❑ Infection
- ❑ Puncture of the heart

DEFINITION

Temporary pacemaker implantation is a common procedure where a pacemaker is inserted just under the skin in the chest with wires attached to the heart.

Temporary pacing is used in emergent or elective situations that require limited, short-term spacing.

PATIENT PREPARATION FOR PACEMAKER IMPLANTATION

- ❏ Assessment of the pacemaker function
- ❏ Assess the heart rate
- ❏ Assess the P wave and QRS complex immediately in cardiac monitor
- ❏ Assess the maintenance of system integrity

STEPS OF PROCEDURE AND RATIONALE

Steps	Rationale
❏ Identify the patient	
❏ Explain the procedure to the patient and family that there will be sensation of discomfort with external spacing	❏ To gain cooperation of client
❏ Get informed consent from the patient or relatives	❏ It protects from health care worker from legalities relating to procedure
❏ Remove dentures, jewelry and contact lens	❏ Removing dentures prevent trauma to the patient
❏ Shave area depending upon site of selection	❏ To reduce the risk for infection
❏ Provide clean gloves	❏ Reduce risk of infection
❏ Start good IV access with heparin lock	❏ To maintain a patent IV line throughout the procedure
❏ Record ECG before procedure and obtain the rhythm strip	❏ Help in comparison after procedure
❏ Administer premedication and send patient to cardiac catheterization lab with patient's chart, X-ray film, lab forms, and ECG rhythm strip	❏ Give information about patient's baseline data
❏ Reassure the patient before procedure	❏ Provide psychological support
❏ Place patient on his back on the procedure table.	
❏ After proper position is provided, the patient will be connected to a cardiac monitor that records the electrical activity of the heart and monitors the heart during the procedure using small adhesive electrodes. Vital signs should be checked during the procedure	❏ It helps us to know the condition of the heart
❏ Large electrode pads will be placed on the front and back of the chest	❏ To get proper electrical impulse
❏ Before the procedure give sedative medication to the patient through intravenously. However, patient will likely remain awake during the procedure	❏ It helps in cooperation of the patient
❏ The pacemaker insertion site will be cleansed with antiseptic soap	❏ To reduce the chance of infection

Contd…

Pacemaker Implantation Procedure

Steps	Rationale
❑ A sterile towel and a sheet will be placed around this area	❑ To make the sterile field
❑ A local anesthetic will be injected into the skin at the insertion site	❑ To reduce pain
❑ Once the anesthetic has taken effect, the physician will make a small incision at the insertion site	❑ To introduce the pacemaker
❑ A sheath, or introducer, is inserted into a blood vessel, usually under the collarbone. The sheath is a plastic tube through which the pacer lead wire will be inserted into the blood vessel and advanced into the heart	❑ To provide electrical impulse
❑ When the catheter is introduced into the vein, alligator clip can be used to connect the exposed tip of the catheter to a cardiac monitor. Larger P waves can be seen as the catheter passes through the atrium and large QRS complex can be seen when catheter is in ventricles. The stimulus and sensitivity are set as per cardiologist order	❑ Monitor the progression of catheter through the heart
❑ The electrode is taped or sutured at insertion site	❑ For better placement of the electrode
❑ Documentation of the procedure: ❑ Date, time of insertion, type of wire inserted and location of insertion ❑ Date and time of initiation of pacing ❑ Pacemaker settings ❑ ECG monitoring strip recordings before and after pacing	❑ For the nurse's record

POSTPROCEDURE CARE

❑ Check vital signs frequently.
❑ Check for the heart rhythm and emotional reaction to procedure.
❑ Monitor battery and control setting.

PERMANANT PACEMAKER IMPLANTATION

DEFINITION

Permanent pacemaker implantation is a procedure in which pacemaker is implanted surgically in the deltopectoral pouch when conduction defect is irreversible.

The implantation of the permanent pacemaker is done in operating room or in the cath lab under fluoroscopic control.

PURPOSES

❑ To transmit impulses from sinus node to ventricles.
❑ To generate impulse spontaneously.
❑ To maintain primary control of pacing function of heart.

INDICATIONS

When a chronic, recurrent conduction or impulse formation disturbance exists in the cardiac conduction system such as:

- Sick sinus syndrome
- Symptomatic sinus bradycardia.
- Atrial fibrillation with a slow ventricular response.
- Complete atrioventricular block (third-degree AV block).
- Chronotropic incompetence (inability to increase the heart rate to match a level of exercise).

COMPLICATIONS

Pacemaker Malfunction

- Failure to output (no pacing spike)
- Failure to capture
- Oversensing
- Undersensing
- Lead dislodgment
- Interference
- Diaphragmatic stimulation

Operative Failures

- Pneumothorax
- Hematoma
- Venous thrombosis
- Pericarditis
- Cardiac perforation
- Skin erosion
- Infection
- Wound dehiscence
- Air embolism
- Subcutaneous emphysema
- Nerve injury
- Thoracic duct injury
- Pain
- Subclavian arterial puncture with hemothorax

Late Complications

- High thresholds
- Lead failure
- Diaphragmatic stimulation
- Infection
- Skin erosion
- Battery depletion
- Loose setscrew
- Pacemaker syndrome
- Venous thrombosis
- Pain

Pacemaker Implantation Procedure

ARTICLES REQUIRED AND THEIR PURPOSES

Articles	Purposes
❑ Electronic cardiac monitor	❑ To monitor cardiac rhythm
❑ Pace maker	❑ To implant pacemaker
❑ Cardiac catheter	❑ To insert catheter
A clean tray containing:	
❑ 1 forceps	❑ To hold the catheter
❑ 1 scissors	❑ To cut the pacemaker wire
❑ 1 retractors	❑ To retract the skin
❑ 1 scalpel blade	❑ To cut the site of insertion
❑ Antiseptic solution	❑ To reduce infection
❑ Local anesthetic agent	❑ To reduce pain
❑ Dynaplast	❑ To cover the site
❑ Resuscitation equipment	❑ For any emergency

STEPS OF PROCEDURE AND RATIONALE

Permanent

Steps	Rationale
❑ Identify the patient	
❑ Explain the procedure and purpose to the patient and family and explain him how he has to cooperate	❑ To gain cooperation of client
❑ Get informed consent	❑ To follow legal process
❑ Explain about need for NBM for 8–10 hours prior to procedure	❑ To prepare for the procedure
❑ Shave following area: ○ Anterior chest from neck to umbilicus ○ Nape of neck to join of back ○ Both arms and axilla	❑ To reduce infection and easy insertion of pacemaker
❑ Remove dentures, jewelry and contact lens	❑ To minimize the electrical contact
❑ Provide clean gloves	❑ Reduce risk of infection
❑ Start good IV access with heparin lock	❑ To maintain electrolyte balance
❑ Record ECG before procedure and obtain the rhythm strip	❑ Help in comparison after procedure
❑ Administer premedication and send patient to cardiac catheterization lab with patient's chart, X-ray film, lab forms, and ECG rhythm strip	❑ Give information about patient's baseline data
❑ Reassure the patient before the procedure	❑ Provide psychological support

Contd…

Principles and Procedures of NURSING FOUNDATIONS

Steps	Rationale
❑ Documentation of the procedure: ○ Date, time of insertion, type of wire inserted and location of insertion ○ Date and time of initiation of pacing ○ Pacemaker settings ○ ECG monitoring strip recordings before and after pacing/pacemaker insertion ○ Vital signs and hemodynamic parameters before, during and after procedure ○ Patient tolerance, comfort level and related interventions ○ Status of skin integrity ○ Medications administered ○ Complications and interventions	❑ For nurse's record

Points to Remember

- ❑ Advice the client to have pacemaker checked every 3 months.
- ❑ Battery replacement should be done between 5 and 15 years (average is 6–7 years).
- ❑ Avoid prolonged contact/exposure with electrical devices or devices with strong magnetic fields such as:
  - ○ Cell phones—may have in shirt pocket if cell phone is turned off
  - ○ MP3 players—wear on right arm
  - ○ Microwaves
  - ○ High-tension wires
  - ○ Metal detectors
- ❑ Stay 2 feet away from industrial welders and electrical generators.
- ❑ No MRI, shock-wave lithotripsy, electrocauterization to stop bleeding during surgery
- ❑ Wear a medical identification tag.
- ❑ Avoid full-contact sports.

Pacemaker Implantation Procedure

NOTES

CHAPTER 32

Assisting in Cardiac Catheterization

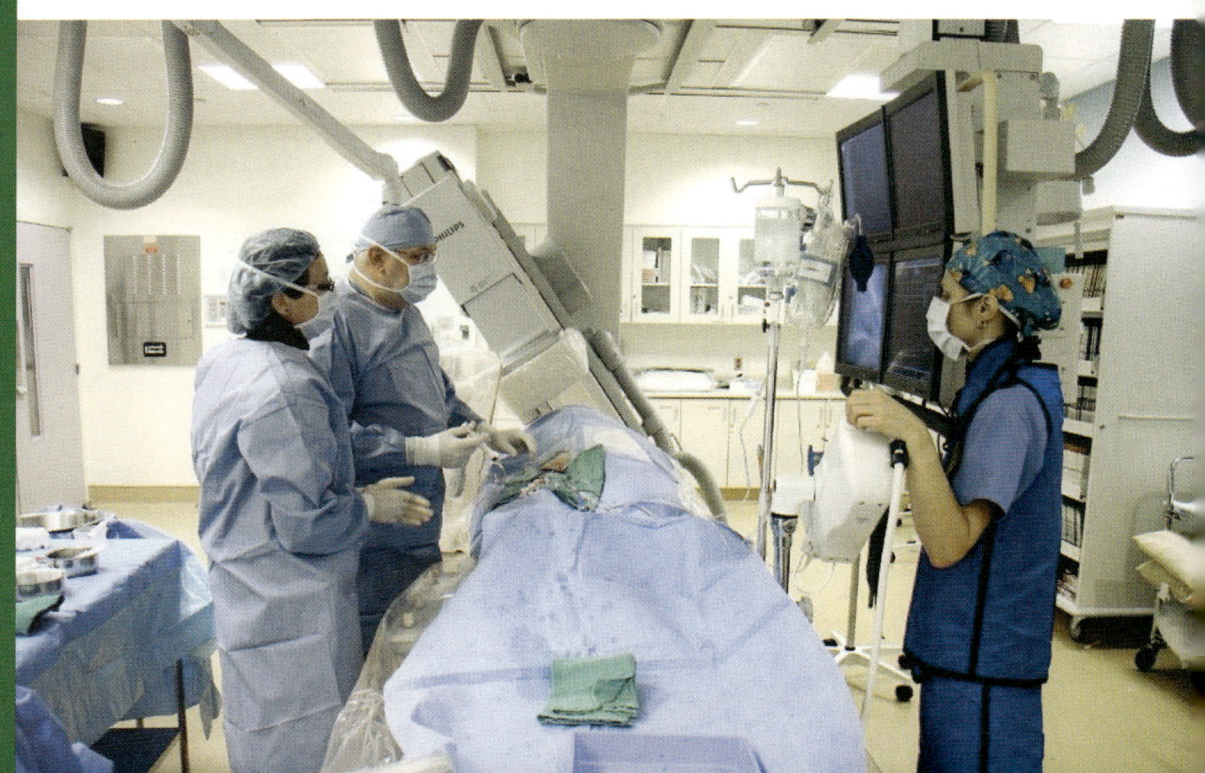

DEFINITION

An invasive diagnostic procedure in which one or more catheters are introduced into heart and selected blood vessels to measure pressures and to determine oxygen saturation in the various heart chambers. The procedure is carried out in cardiac catheterization lab.

PURPOSES

- ❑ To assess patency of coronary arteries.
- ❑ To decide on appropriate treatment e.g. PTCA/CABG (Percutaneous coronary intervention/coronary after bypass grafting) if atherosclerosis is present.
- ❑ To measure pressures in various chambers of the heart.
- ❑ To obtain blood samples for measurement of hematocrit and oxygen saturation.
- ❑ To confirm diagnosis of heart disease and to determine the extent to which the disease has affected structure and functions of heart.
- ❑ To obtain clear picture of cardiac anatomy prior to heart surgery.
- ❑ To determine cardiac output.
- ❑ To obtain endocardial biopsies.
- ❑ To allow infusion of fibrinolytic agents directly into the occluded coronary artery to restore coronary blood flow.

RIGHT HEART CATHETERIZATION

Passing a radiopaque catheter through internal jugular/subclavian/femoral vein into the right atrium, right ventricle and pulmonary artery.

LEFT HEART CATHETERIZATION

Insertion of a catheter through brachial artery or femoral artery to aorta and left ventricle. It can also be performed transparently from right atrium into left atrium and then left ventricle.

ARTICLES REQUIRED AND THEIR PURPOSES

Articles	Purposes
❑ Cardiac monitor	❑ To monitor cardiac condition
❑ Pressure monitoring device	❑ To assess the pressure within the heart
❑ Fluoroscope	❑ To visualize heart and arteries
❑ Sterile radiopaque cardiac catheters	❑ To insert in the heart through the vein
❑ Radiopaque dye	❑ To visualize arteries and vein
❑ Sterile linen for draping	❑ To avoid soiling of patient garments
❑ Cleaning solutions	❑ To minimize infection at the puncture site
❑ Sterile gloves	
❑ Cardiac catheterization pack	
❑ Cut down set	
❑ Scalpel blade	
❑ Emergency articles	
❑ Sterile gown	❑ To reduce cross infection
❑ Local anesthetic agent	❑ To reduce pain
❑ Sterile syringes and needles	❑ Sterile syringes to insert the dye

CONTRAINDICATIONS

- ❑ Pregnancy because of risk of radioactive iodine crossing the blood placental barrier
- ❑ Cardiomyopathy
- ❑ Severe dysrhythmias
- ❑ Uncontrolled congestive heart failure
- ❑ Patient allergic to local anesthesia, iodine or radiopaque contrast material
- ❑ Bleeding disorders

STEPS OF PROCEDURE AND RATIONALE

Steps	Rationale
❑ Assess patient's knowledge of procedure and explain procedure to she patient	❑ To allay anxiety and ensures cooperation of the patient
❑ Assess vital signs including peripheral pulses, heart and lung sounds and body weight	❑ Provides baseline data for comparison of findings during and after the procedure
❑ Determine whether right or left heart is being studied	❑ Enables nurse to anticipate patient teaching needs and postprocedure interventions
❑ Assess whether patient has signed consent forms	❑ Both types of procedures usually require. Informed consent to reduce legal risk
❑ Assess time of last ingested fluid or food. Patient should be NPO for 6–8 hours before the procedure	❑ Prevents possible aspiration since patient is sedated for the procedure. Excessive hydration causes dilution of the contrast medium which makes structures more difficult to visualize
❑ Assess if patient is allergic to iodine dye. If so, notify the cardiologist or radiologist	❑ An iodine based radiopaque contrast medium may be used during the procedure. However, a hypoallergenic contrast medium is more frequently used
❑ Assess the blood count, platelets and prothrombin time, electrolytes, BUN, creatinine levels etc., prior to the procedures	❑ Abnormal findings might contraindicate the procedure since hemorrhage or renal failure may occur
❑ Review physician's order for preprocedural medications ○ Atropine (contraindicated in glaucoma) ○ Benadryl ○ Sedative	❑ Decreases or prevents bradycardia, caused by vagal stimulation and decreases oral secretions
❑ Mark digital pulses	❑ Enables easy reference after procedure
❑ Instruct the patient to empty his/her bladder	❑ Ensures that patient will be comfortable during procedure
❑ Wash hands and prepare area as per surgical procedure	❑ Reduces transmission of microorganisms
❑ Don mask, goggles, sterile gown, cap and gloves. Drape patient with sterile drapes	❑ Protects nurse from risk of infection. Maintains surgical asepsis
❑ Assist in anesthetizing the skin overlying the arterial puncture site	❑ Provides local anesthesia to areas of incision or puncture site
❑ Assist in performing needle puncture of artery inserting ❑ Guide wire through needle and threading angiographic catheter Cardiologist advances catheter to desired artery or cardiac chamber and injects contrast medium	❑ Permits access to artery and prevents coiling of catheter in artery ❑ Permits radiographic visualization of structure, aneurysms, occlusions or anomalies.

Contd…

Assisting in Cardiac Catheterization

Steps	Rationale
❑ Explain the patient that he will experience a feeling of heat, ○ Flushing of face and a desire to cough during dye injection and X-ray films will be taken rapidly at this time	❑ Permits radiographic records of visualization of dye through artery as well as any abnormalities present. Adequate explanation reduces anxiety of patient
❑ Physician withdraws catheter after the entire procedure is over. Apply pressure to puncture site for at least 10–20 minutes. Assess puncture site for hematoma formation at site and increase in pain/tenderness	❑ Pressure on puncture site promotes clotting and prevents bleeding
❑ Apply pressure dressing over puncture site	❑ To prevent bleeding
❑ Monitor vital signs, apical and peripheral pulses, auscultate heart and lungs after cardiac catheterization every 15 minutes until stable and compare with baseline values	❑ Verifies patient's physiologic status and evaluates effect of procedure on physiologic functions
❑ Assess the patient for possible delayed reaction to iodine dye like dyspnea, hives, tachycardia or rash	❑ Reaction may occur up to few hours after injection of dye
❑ Assess postprocedure laboratory values such as blood count, prothrombin time, electrolytes, blood count and creatinine	❑ Changes in laboratory values many indicate the onset of complications
❑ Instruct the patient about strict bed rest for 12–24 hours and to keep affected extremity straight for 12 hours	❑ To prevent bleeding
❑ Encourage fluid intake	❑ To promote excretion of dye
❑ Record type of cardiac catheterization done and patient's tolerance of the procedure	❑ Note in the documents patient's response to invasive procedure
❑ Record type of dressing, amount and type of drainage and presence of pain or discomfort	❑ To provide baseline data for determining patient's progress

Points to Remember

❑ Make the patient to lie in supine position in the recovery room.
❑ Apply pressure over the puncture site to reduce the bleeding.

CHAPTER 33

Assisting in Application of Plaster Cast

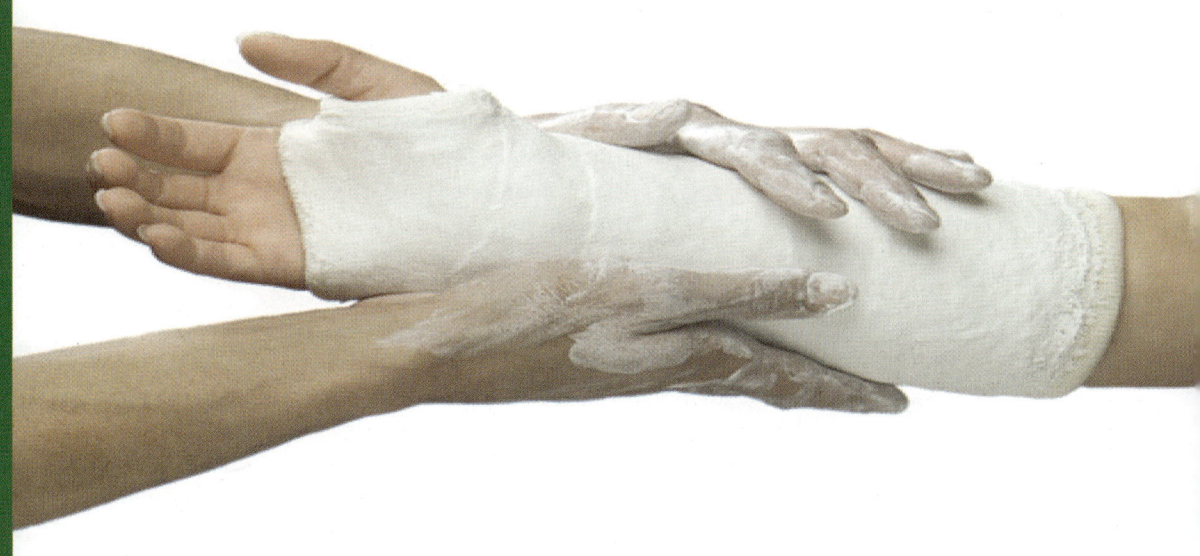

DEFINITION

A plaster cast slab or splint is applied in broken bones of upper or lower extremity. Plaster can be applied for a temporary period while waiting for definitive treatment of an injured part.

PURPOSES

- ❏ To immobilize the body part in specific position
- ❏ To apply equal pressure on soft tissue
- ❏ To correct and prevent deformity
- ❏ To provide support for weak joints
- ❏ To immobilize a reduced fracture.

TYPES

- ❏ Short arm cast (wrist plaster)
- ❏ Long arm cast (above elbow plaster)
- ❏ Arm cylinder cast
- ❏ Short leg cast (below knee plaster)
- ❏ Leg cylinder cast
- ❏ Shoulder spica cast
- ❏ Minerva cast
- ❏ Bivalved cast

ARTICLES REQUIRED AND THEIR PURPOSES

Articles	Purposes
❏ Plaster bandages	❏ To roll bandages over the plaster cast
❏ Stockinette	❏ To reduce skin irritation
❏ Short trimming knife	❏ To cut the plaster cast
❏ Scissors	❏ To cut the bandages
❏ Dressing supplies	❏ To cover the plaster cast
❏ Measuring tape	❏ To measure the length of the plaster
❏ Protective sheet	❏ To protect the plaster cast
❏ Plastic apron	❏ To prevent soiling of the cloths
❏ Gloves	❏ To prevent cross infection and to protect the hands
❏ Newspaper	❏ To make rest the plaster cast
❏ Fracture table	❏ Helps to position the patient properly
❏ Shaving set	❏ To remove the unwanted hairs or clean the site of fracture

STEPS OF PROCEDURE AND RATIONALE

Steps	Rationale
❏ Asses the patient's health status, including conditions affecting wound healing	❏ Patient's health status depends on healing of tissues enclosed by cast
❏ Explain to the patient the pressure and procedure of cast application as per his level of understanding	❏ Relieves patient's anxiety and helps the nurse to determine whether additional information is needed

Contd…

Steps	Rationale
❑ Assess condition of tissues to be in the cast including circulation to the extremities. If the skin breaks down or bruising rash and irritation may contain in subcutaneous tissue	❑ Determines need for additional skin care before cast application
❑ Assess the level of pain of the patient	❑ All types of fracture are painful
❑ Protective sheet is used to protect the patient's cloths	❑ To prevent soiling of bed sheet
❑ Administer analgesics 20–30 minutes before the application of cast	❑ To reduce pain during cast application
❑ Wash hands and don gloves	❑ To reduce transmission of microorganism
❑ Position the patient: Patient can be lying sitting or standing depending upon the body part to be cast	❑ Fractured part to optimally positioned for the application of cast
❑ Prepare skin for the cast if necessary which involves cleansing with soap and water, changing the dressing and rimming or shaving long hairs	❑ Reduces complications to underlying tissues after casting
❑ Place stockinette over the skin where casting material will be applied (Fig. 1)	❑ Reduces skin irritation

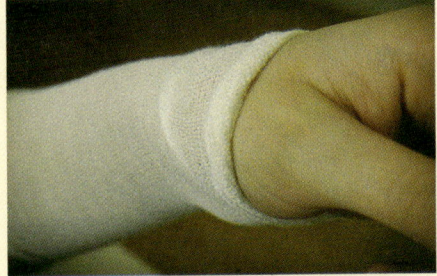

FIG. 1: Placing stockinette over the skin

❑ Wrap the site with cast padding (Fig. 2)

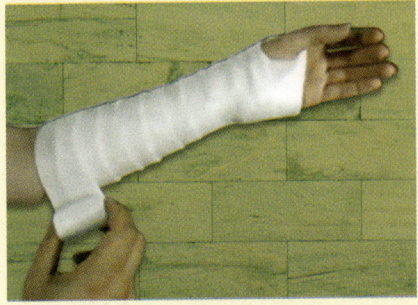

FIG. 2: Padding the cast site

❑ Depending on the type of cast material following can be applied:
  ○ Hold plaster roll under water in a casting bucket or plastic basin until bubbles stop (Fig. 3). Then squeeze slightly and hand over to person applying cast
  ○ Submerge synthetic cast roll in lukewarm water for 15 seconds and squeeze to remove excess water.
  ○ Hold the body parts or the parts to be put in cast in position requested for applying the cast.

Contd…

Assisting in Application of Plaster Cast

Steps	Rationale
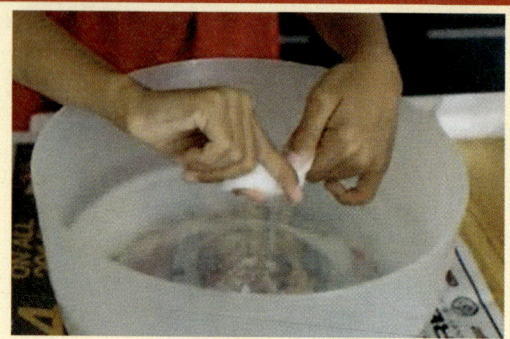 **FIG. 3:** Holding plaster roll under water	
❑ Continue to apply dampened rolls of plaster to hold parts as necessary until cast is finished (Fig. 4) 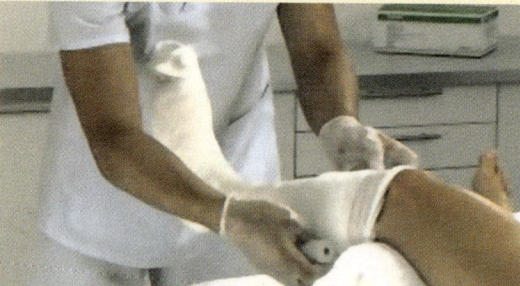 **FIG. 4:** Applying plaster rolls	❑ Plaster should be of adequate thickness to give strength to cast
❑ Assist with finishing the cast by folding stockinette or other padding down the outer edge of cast to provide smooth edge to cast. Damp plaster is then rolled over padding to hold it securely outside cast (Fig. 5) 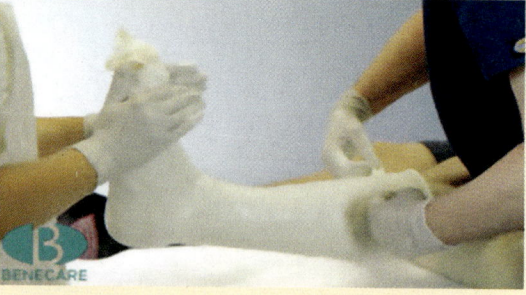 **FIG. 5:** Finishing of the cast application	❑ Smooth edges reduces the chances of irritation finishing cast with stockinette provides smooth edges. It is required when cast is dry.
❑ Using scissors trim plaster roll around thumb, finger or toes as necessary	❑ Cast should be snug but should not constrict joint movement or circulation
❑ Depending on the tissues to be cast follow this: ○ Place damp cast on cloth covered pillows to prevent deformation or pressure points as plaster gets set. ○ Handle the damp plaster only with the palm of the hand	❑ Pillows or soft areas prevent cast from hardening in undesirable position. Handling plaster cast with fingers can cause indentation

Contd…

Steps	Rationale
❑ Remove your gloves and assist with transfer of patient to the stretcher or wheel chair for return to the bed	❑ Safety require support of pillows side rails restraints, and sufficient personnel to support patient and cast
❑ Clean equipment used, return to usual place, discard the used material and wash hands	❑ Articles can be used for next time or next patient and reduces transmission of infection
❑ Explain purposes of exposure for faster drying use elevation if required. Apply ice bags if ordered. Use fans or hair dryer and set to cool setting to facilitate drying	❑ Cast must dry outside as well as from inside , for through drying of the cast is elevation is required and applying ice will reduce edema
❑ Turn the patient every 2–3 hours	❑ To prevent one area of cast receiving continuous pressure
❑ Observe the patient for the signs of pain and anxiety hyperventilation of air tachycardia or increased BP	❑ There are signs of cast syndrome which may occur when body cast is applied
❑ Neurovascular assessment: ○ Observe the color of the tissue below to the cast applied ○ Observe to the edema distal to the cast ○ Feel temperature of tissues above and below the cast ○ Palpate the pulse of the distal area of the extremity record pulse presence and strength ○ Ask the patient to move parts distal to the cast in ROM if possible perform passive ROM in these joints	❑ It helps to determine circulation of tissue. ❑ Pink color indicates arterial pressure is normal ❑ Edema results from trauma or venous stasis ❑ Warmth over the tissues indicate proper blood supply to the area ❑ Weak or absent of pulse indicates decreased circulation to the area ❑ ROM is possible within limitation
❑ Record application of the cast and condition of the skin and circulation status.	
❑ Record patient's ability and inability to do activity of daily life (ADL), specific requirement of care	❑ Independence is valued for continuity of care and self-care

COMPLICATIONS

❑ Impaired blood flow
❑ Nerve damage
❑ Tissue necrosis and infection
❑ Volkmann's ischemic contracture
❑ Cast syndrome
❑ Complication due to immobility.

Points to Remember

❑ It should be informed properly to the patient that sensation of heat may occur at the time of drying of the plaster cast.
❑ Plaster cast should not be applied over the open wound.

Assisting in Application of Plaster Cast

NOTES

CHAPTER 34

Skeletal Traction

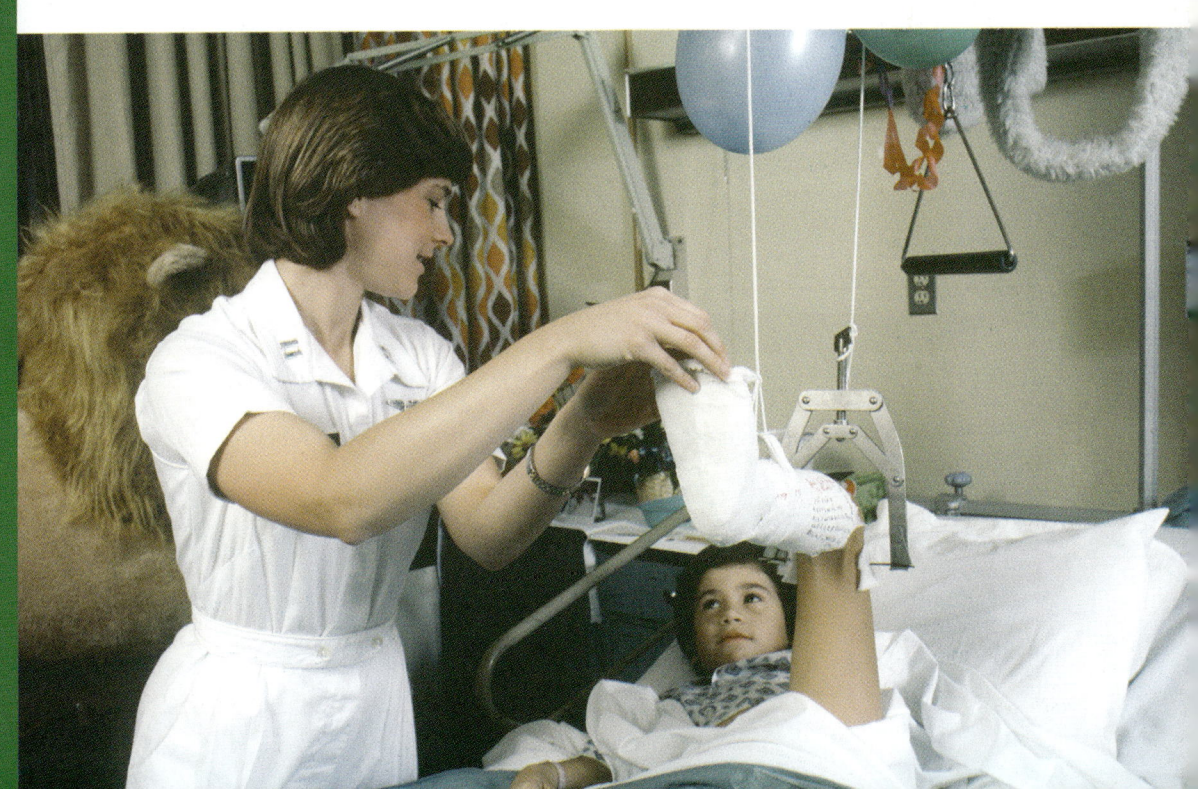

DEFINITION

Skeletal traction is accomplished by introducing a metal tongs wire or metal pins (Steinmann pins) or metal tongs under strict aseptic technique through the bones beneath the fracture. The traction is applied directly to the bone by use of a metal pin or wire that is inserted through the bone distal to the fracture.

SITES OF SKELETAL TRACTION

- ❑ Below the olecranon process
- ❑ Below the olecranon together with a pin through the distal ends of the radius and the ulna
- ❑ Through the middle three metacarpals
- ❑ Through the distal phalanx of the fingers
- ❑ Through the supracondylar area of the femur
- ❑ Through the upper end of the tibia
- ❑ Through the lower end of the tibia and fibula
- ❑ Through the ossicles
- ❑ Through the distal phalanx of the toes
- ❑ Skull traction

TYPES OF SKELETAL TRACTION

- ❑ Balanced skeletal traction with a Thomas splint and a flexion piece.
- ❑ Proximal tibial traction with balanced suspension.

INDICATIONS

- ❑ Fracture of femur
- ❑ Fractures of humerus
- ❑ Fracture of tibia
- ❑ Fracture of cervical spine

CONTRAINDICATION OF SKELETAL TRACTION

- ❑ Bone infection or skin infection/rash through which wire/pins are to be passed
- ❑ Hematoma of fracture site

STEPS OF PROCEDURE AND RATIONALE

Steps	Rationale
❑ Explain the procedure of skeletal traction to the patient	❑ To get cooperation and written permission from the patient for surgery
❑ Prepare the skin as per requirement of specific traction like	❑ To prevent infection
❑ Tibia–shave waistline to ankle of the affected leg including private parts	❑ Skin preparation prevents the growth of micro-organisms
❑ Fracture of pelvis—shave the skin from hip to knee including private parts	
❑ Fracture of cervical spine—shaving of complete skull should be done	
❑ Check for the site of specific skeletal traction should be applied	❑ To ensure correct site of skeletal traction

GENERAL STEPS OF PREOPERATIVE CARE OF THE PATIENT AND RATIONALE

Steps	Rationale
❑ Keep the client fasting for 6 hours before surgery	❑ Helps to prevent regurgitation and aspiration of food during surgery
❑ Take consent	❑ It helps in legal aspects
❑ Give soap and water enema or proctoclysis enema on the day of surgery	❑ It helps to empty the bowels and prevents infection
❑ Check vital signs before sending the patient to OT	❑ It provides baseline data. Normal vital signs indicate normal function of vital organs

STEPS OF POSTOPERATIVE CARE OF THE PATIENT WITH APPLICATION OF SKELETAL TRACTION AND RATIONALE

Steps	Rationale
❑ Pain due to surgical insertion of pin or wires, fracture and immobilization with traction	❑ Assessment of pain characteristic, location intensity and duration, assure the patient ❑ Provide a comfortable position ❑ Administer analgesics as per doctor's order
❑ Impaired physical mobility related to traction application and knowledge deficit about the importance of and why physical immobilization is required	❑ Provide correct body alignment ❑ Injured part or the position of the patient should not be disturbed ❑ Maintain balance traction over the fragments of bones. Place all joints through the range of motion ❑ Encourage the patient through the isometric leg exercise
❑ High risk for injury related to traction	❑ Ensure that weight hangs freely from pulleys ❑ Ensure that knots in the rope do not catch in the pulleys

Precautions to be Taken during Application of the Skeletal Traction

❑ Wires and pins are not inserted through joints
❑ They are inserted so that they only penetrate skin subcutaneous tissues and bones
❑ They are not inserted in the skin that is infected
❑ Avoid unsterile techniques while inserting

Removal of Skeletal Traction

When skeletal traction is to be removed, prepare the skin around the pin site according to the physician instructions
❑ Depressing the skin around the wire end
❑ Cutting the wire beneath the skin surface
❑ Pulling the wire from the opposite side
❑ Cutting one end of the pin prevents the bone from exposure to the contaminated end of the pin.

Complication of Skeletal Traction

❑ Foot drop
❑ Bed sore
❑ Renal calculi

Skeletal Traction

- Constipation
- Urinary tract-infection UTI
- Malnourished
- Pulmonary embolism
- Volkmann's ischemic contractures

Points to Remember

- Proper alignment should be checked.
- Weight should accurate.

CHAPTER 35

Skin Traction

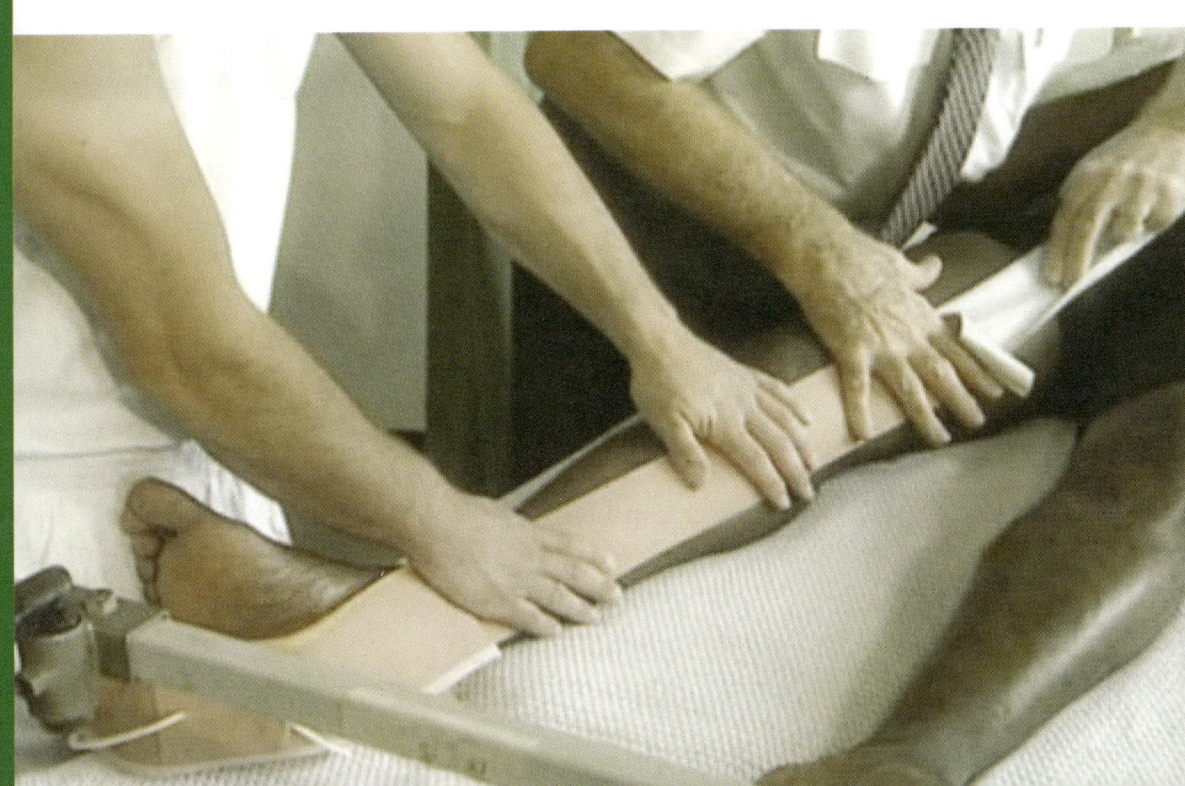

DEFINITION

Skin traction is defined as a non-surgical procedure which indirectly applies traction on an underlying structure, e.g. muscles. Skin traction is achieved by clinging wide bands of adhesives to the skin and applying weights to those bands.

INDICATIONS

- ❑ Muscle spasm and pain
- ❑ Prior to surgery in the treatment of hip fracture and femoral shaft fracture
- ❑ Pelvic and cervical traction for back disorders or injuries
- ❑ Fracture in children

TYPES

- ❑ **Buck's extension:** Buck's extension is a form of skin traction in which the pull is exerted in one plane when partial or temporary immobilization is desirable. It can be applied to one leg (unilateral) or both (bilateral) as per the indication or need of the client.
- ❑ **Bryant's traction:** Bryant's traction which is a skin traction, is applied to both lower limbs. It can be used to reduce fractures of the femur in children under 6 years.
- ❑ **Russell's traction:** Russell's traction may be used in the treatment of fracture of hip shaft of femur, tibia and fibula. It may be applied as skeletal traction also.

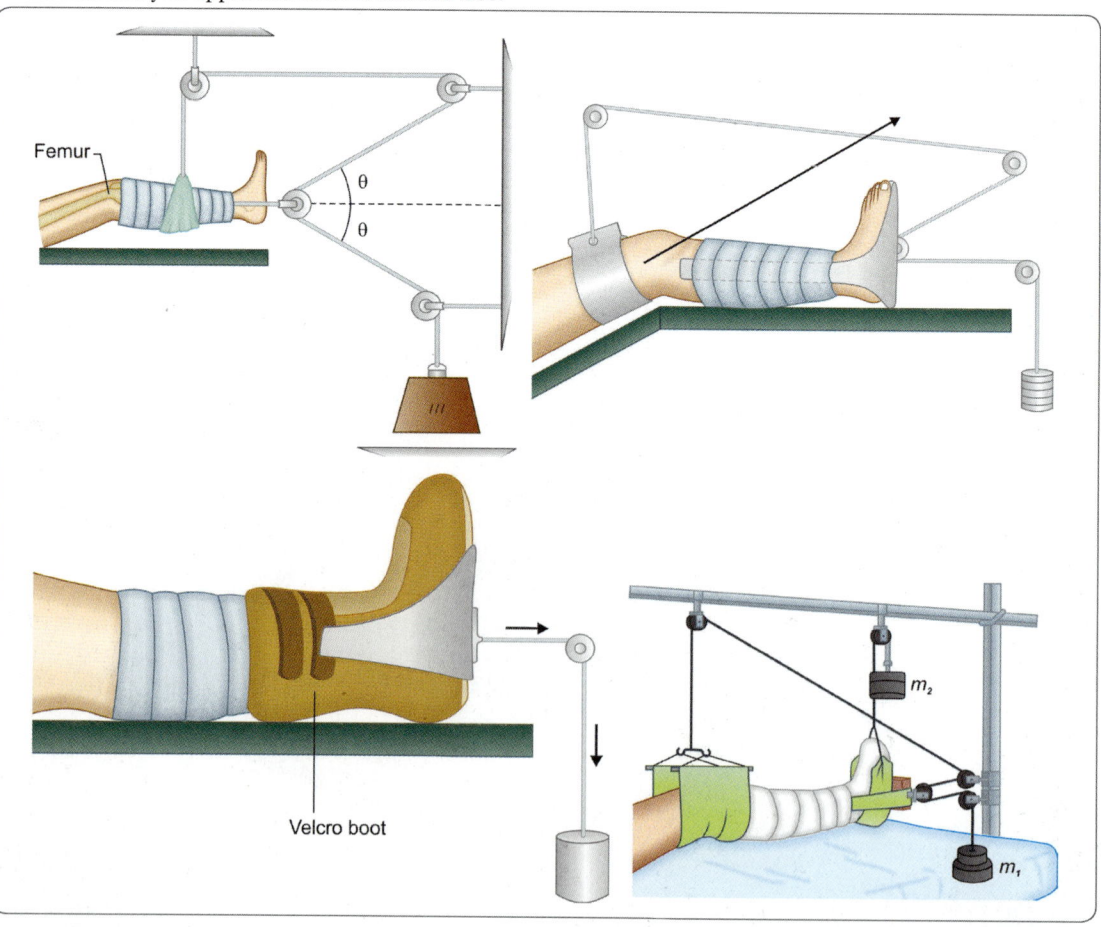

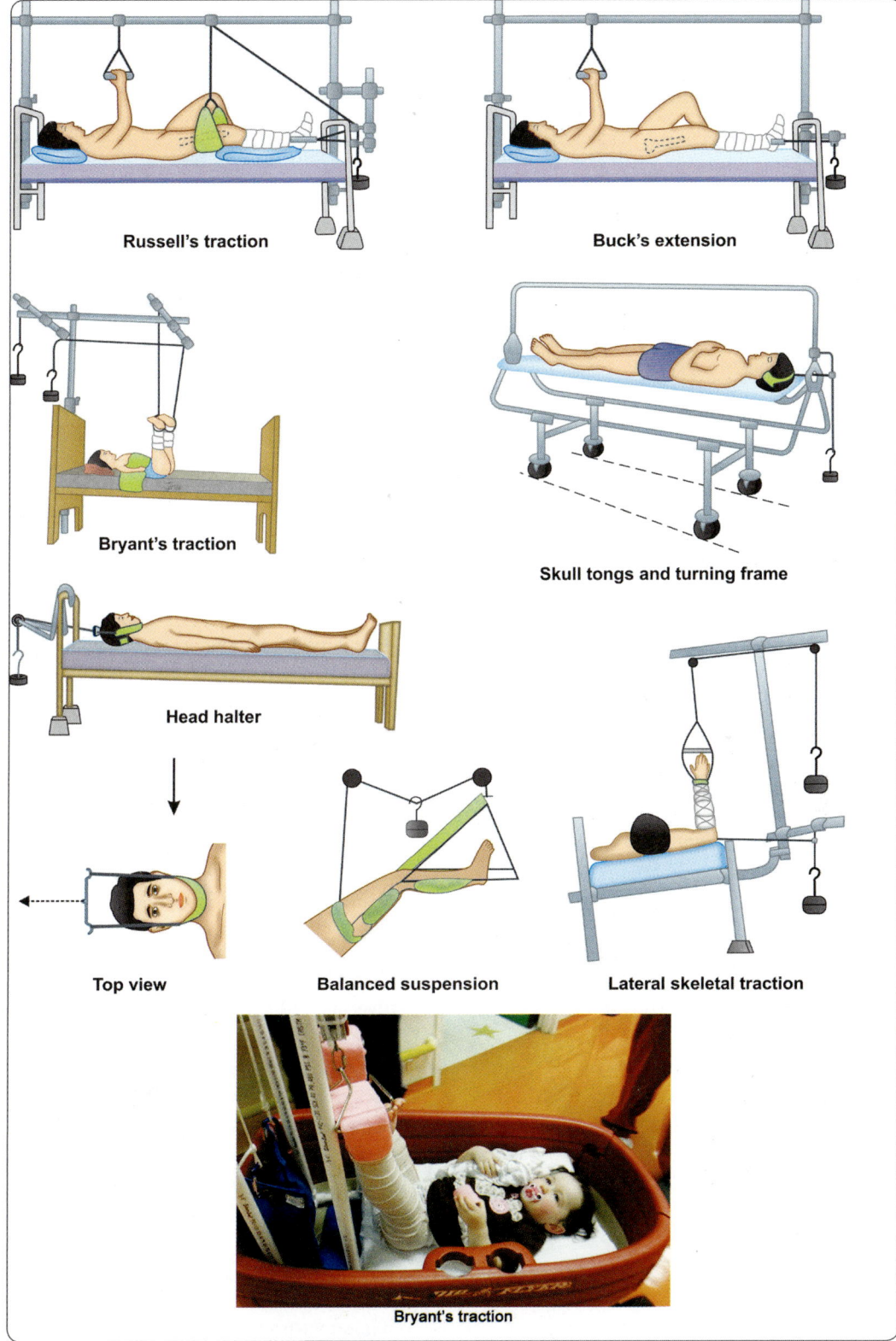

Russell's traction

Buck's extension

Bryant's traction

Skull tongs and turning frame

Head halter

Top view

Balanced suspension

Lateral skeletal traction

Bryant's traction

Skin Traction

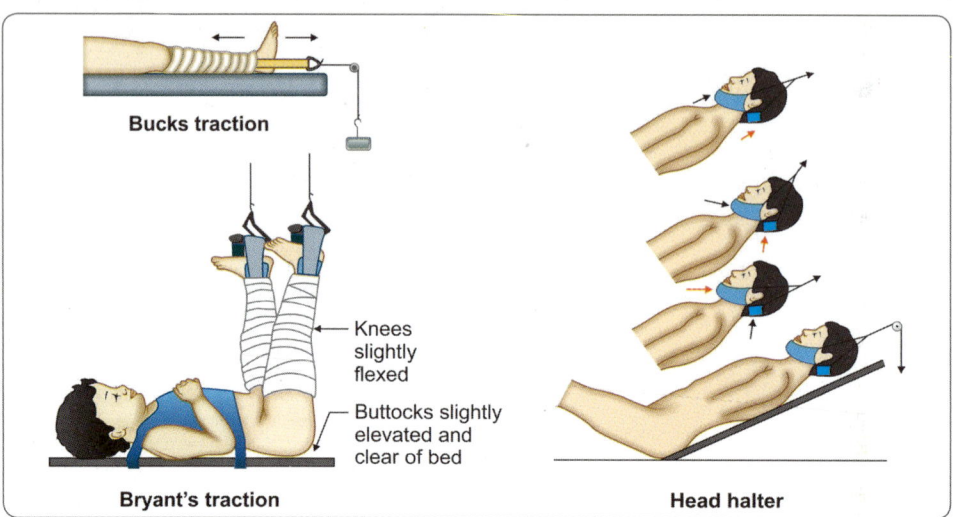

Bucks traction

Bryant's traction

Knees slightly flexed

Buttocks slightly elevated and clear of bed

Head halter

GENERAL INSTRUCTIONS FOR APPLICATION OF SKIN TRACTION

Preliminary Assessment

- ❑ Check the patient's name, bed no, and identification data.
- ❑ Check the nature of the patient's injury and his/her general condition.
- ❑ Check the purpose of the traction.
- ❑ Check the doctor's order for the type of traction to be applied, its duration amount of weight and movements allowed.
- ❑ Check the integrity of the skin where the traction is to be applied.

ARTICLES REQUIRED AND THEIR PURPOSES

Articles	Purposes
❑ Adhesive plaster (full length)	❑ To apply on the skin for use as a traction strip
❑ Scissors	❑ To cut the plaster
❑ Tincture benzoin	❑ To promote adhesion of the adhesive plaster and to maintain integrity of the skin
❑ Spreader (rectangular wooden piece) with a small hole in the center	❑ To keep the traction strips off the malleolus and to apply the weight
❑ Roller bandage	❑ To cover and secure the traction tapes
❑ Traction rope (strong)	❑ To tie and apply the weights
❑ Sterile cotton balls in a container	❑ To apply tincture of benzoin
❑ A kidney tray and a paper bag	❑ To discard the cotton swab after application
❑ Cross bars and camps	❑ To fix the pulley in position
❑ Pulleys	❑ To apply the traction freely in the direction as desired
❑ Bed Blocks	❑ To raise the foot end of the bed to apply counter traction
❑ Measuring tape	❑ To measure the length of tape
❑ Weight as ordered	❑ To apply traction
❑ A Balkan frame with a trapeze bed or a firm bed with a mattress	❑ To suspend the cross bars pulleys etc. and also help the patient to lift his body when needed
❑ Thomas splint if ordered	❑ To support the fractured leg

Principles and Procedures of NURSING FOUNDATIONS

Materials Used

Sponge rubber and canvas material are used as adhesive plaster.

STEPS OF PROCEDURE OF BUCK'S EXTENSION SKIN TRACTION AND RATIONALE

Steps	Rationale
❑ Wash and dry hands	❑ Helps in prevention of cross infection
❑ Measure the length of the adhesive tape needed. Measure the length 4" above the knee to the malleolus and add 10" to extend beyond the foot and to cover that spreader and then double it to cover the opposite side of the leg	❑ Correct length of the tape helps in the correct application of the traction and prevents wastage of the adhesive plaster ❑ Correct application of traction helps in reduction of fractured bones
❑ If fixed traction is ordered, limb should be placed in and traction rope is tied to the end of the Thomas splint	❑ Fixed traction will not disturb the alignment of the body. Effective support is provided with the Thomas splint
❑ The spreader is supported in place by the second strip of adhesive which should extend 10"–12" on each side of the wood to prevent adhesion to the malleoli	❑ The second strip fixed to the adhesive surface of the first strip will prevent the plaster from wrinkling. Ensure correct way of application of traction
❑ Apply adhesive strip smoothly without wrinkles on the lateral and medial aspect of the thigh and lower leg. The crest of the tibia and the patella is not covered with the strip	❑ Wrinkles can cause pressure on the skin and cause pressure sores. Care should be taken to protect the bony prominence. Effective application of traction hastens the healing
❑ To apply buck's extension with tape foam rubber padded strips are used on the surface against the skin on each side of the affected leg ❑ A loop of tape about 10–15 cm long is extended beyond the sole of the foot	❑ The rubber padded strips will protect the patient from pressure against the skin and bony prominence

STEPS OF PROCEDURE OF BRYANT'S TRACTION (GALLOW'S TRACTION) AND RATIONALE

Steps	Rationale
❑ Skin traction is applied to both lower limbs. Both legs are suspended vertically with the hip flexed at 90° and the knees are extended. The buttocks are slightly elevated from the mattress.	❑ To reduce fracture of the femur in children of 6 years. As the counter-traction provided by the weight of the trunk is not sufficient, vertical suspension of both the legs in correct, straight alignment provides traction in a proper way. The body weight is used to provide the counter traction. Effective application of traction for children hastens healing of the bone fractures. ❑ Equal traction and counter traction is essential.

STEPS OF PROCEDURE OF THE RUSSELL'S TRACTION AND RATIONALE

Steps	Rationale
❑ The traction is applied in Buck's extension and the sling passes below the knee	❑ It helps to reduce or immobilize hip fracture or the shaft of the femur or tibia plateau. Effective applications of traction hasten the healing of bones in correct union of fractures

Contd…

Skin Traction

Steps	Rationale
❑ Secure the adhesive strips in place for bandaging. The leg bandages must not be so light to interfere with the blood or nerve supply to the limb	❑ Unless fixed with bandages the traction strips should be pulled away from the skin when it is applied
❑ Thread the traction rope to the center of the spreader and pass it through pulleys and apply weight as ordered. The height of the pulley should be adjusted with the center of the spreader to keep rope and pulleys in straight alignment	❑ Equal traction and counter traction is essential for reduction of a bone
❑ Raise the foot end of the bed on bed blocks	❑ To obtain counter traction. Body pulls against weight and acts as counter traction
❑ A cord is attached to the sling and passes up vertically to a pulley on the overhead beam and then passed over several pulleys at the foot of the bed on which the weight is added	❑ Counter traction is supplied by pressure against the ischial tuberosity and the body weight when the foot of the bed is elevated
❑ A foot support with a sling is provided	❑ To prevent foot drop. Disuse of muscle gives a chance of developing contractures

REMOVAL OF THE SKIN TRACTION

At the time of removal of the traction, the patient will probably be found weak and unsteady. Some muscles may become atrophy and orthostatic hypotension may develop in some patients.

It has to be removed slowly as adhesive plaster is sticking to the skin. During removal, wet the plaster with saline and remove the adhesive plaster. Apply coconut oil to the skin and passive exercises and slow massage to be given to the affected extremity.

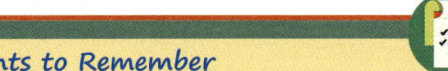

Points to Remember

❑ Do not apply the traction cast too tightly.
❑ Provide a foot support with a sling.

CHAPTER 36

Assisting in Liver Biopsy

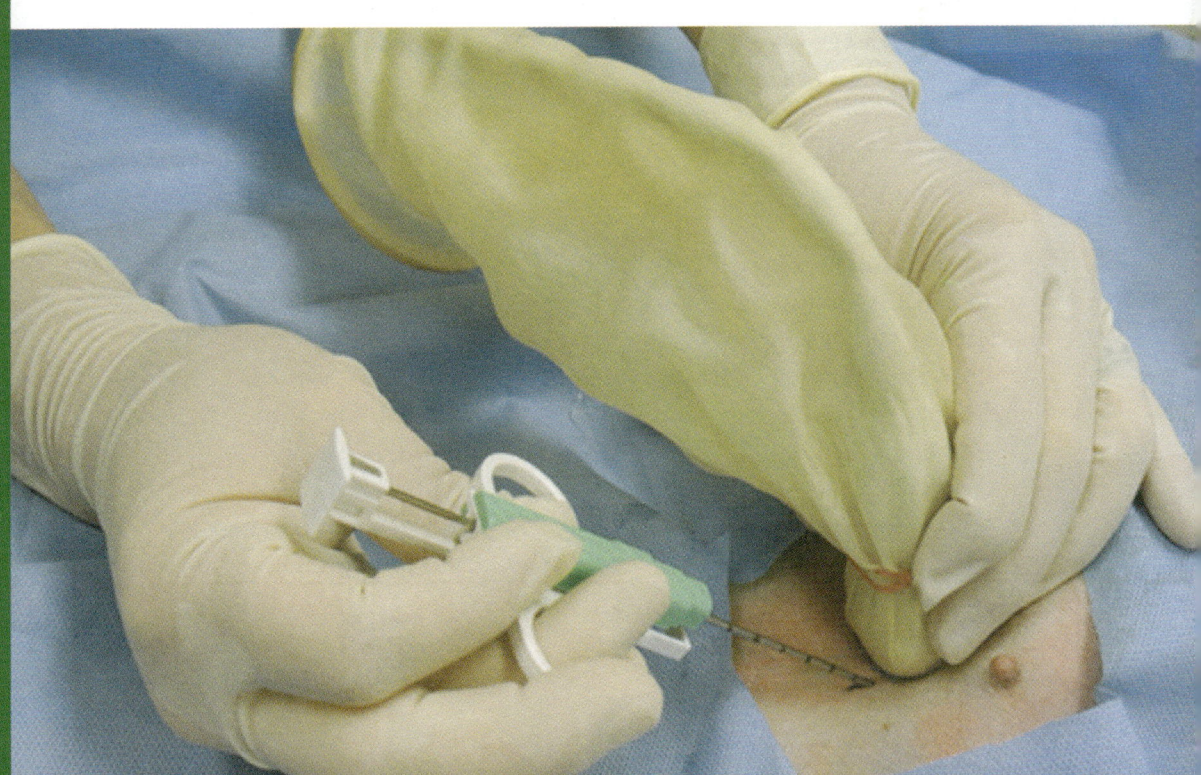

DEFINITION

A biopsy of the liver is a medical procedure in which a small amount of liver tissue is surgically removed so it can be tested in a laboratory.

Assisting in collecting sample of liver tissue by needle aspiration using aseptic technique.

PURPOSES

- ❑ To diagnose any digestive system disorders
- ❑ To diagnose liver disease through histopathology study

INDICATIONS

- ❑ Alcoholic liver disease
- ❑ Autoimmune hepatitis
- ❑ Hepatitis (B, C)
- ❑ Hemochromatosis
- ❑ Nonalcoholic fatty liver disease
- ❑ Primary biliary cirrhosis
- ❑ Primary sclerosing cholangitis
- ❑ Wilson's disease

ARTICLES REQUIRED AND THEIR PURPOSES

Articles	Purposes
A sterile tray containing:	
❑ Sponge holding forceps	❑ To hold the instruments
❑ Syringe 5 mL	
❑ Liver biopsy needle with stilette	
❑ Specimen bottles with cork	❑ To collect the specimen
❑ Bowl	❑ To take cleaning lotion
❑ Aspiration syringe	❑ If aspiration biopsy to be done
❑ Dissecting forceps	
❑ Dressing towels	
❑ Cotton balls, gauze pieces and cotton pads	❑ To clean the site
❑ Gown, gloves and mask	❑ To prevent cross infection
A clean tray containing:	
❑ Mackintosh and towel	❑ To avoid soiling of bed
❑ Kidney tray	❑ To collect the waste
❑ Spirit, tincture benzoin etc.	❑ To clean the site
❑ Lignocaine 2%	❑ To reduce the pain
❑ Adhesive plaster and scissors	❑ To fix the site after procedure
❑ Formalin 10%	❑ To preserve the biopsy specimen

STEPS OF PROCEDURE AND RATIONALE

Steps	Rationale
❏ Explain the procedure to the patient and family and inform them to cooperate	❏ Helps in obtaining cooperation of patient and reduces anxiety
❏ Obtain informed consent form patient	❏ Prevents litigation of staff members
❏ Ensure that patient's coagulation profile is within a normal limit	❏ Prevents bleeding complication during procedure
❏ Check baseline vital signs and records	❏ Helps in obtaining baseline data
❏ Instruct the patient to be on NPO for 6–8 hours before procedure	❏ Prevents entry of food into the lungs and reduces the risk of pneumonia during anesthesia.
❏ Instruct the patient not to take aspirin NSAID, anticoagulant 2 weeks before the procedure	❏ Prevents bleeding tendencies
❏ Administer premedication (analgesia sedation) as per doctor's order	
❏ Provide supine position to the patient or in left lateral position with right arm elevated	❏ This position helps for easy insertion of needle
❏ Shave and clean 8th and 9th intercostals space at the incision site	
❏ Instruct the patient to take deep breath and to hold the breath while the needle is introduced through the intercostals or subcostal tissue into the liver	❏ Avoids puncturing of the diaphragm
❏ The special needle assemble is inserted and is rotated to separate a fragment of tissue and then is withdrawn	
❏ Assist doctor to seal puncture site with tincture benzoin and apply pressure dressing	
❏ Collect the specimen in a sterile container label it and send it to laboratory	
❏ Instruct the patient to lie on his right side	
❏ Record the procedure with date and time and any complication occurred.	❏ Acts as a communication between the staff members

COMPLICATIONS

- ❏ **Immediate complications**
  - ○ Abdominal pain
  - ○ Pneumothorax
  - ○ Injury to stomach, pancreas, small intestine, kidney and diaphragm
- ❏ **Late complications**
  - ○ Hemorrhage
  - ○ Shock and collapse
  - ○ Bile peritonitis

Point to Remember

❏ Avoid intense activity like weight lifting for up to two weeks.

Assisting in Liver Biopsy

NOTES

CHAPTER 37

Assisting with Bone Marrow Aspiration and Biopsy

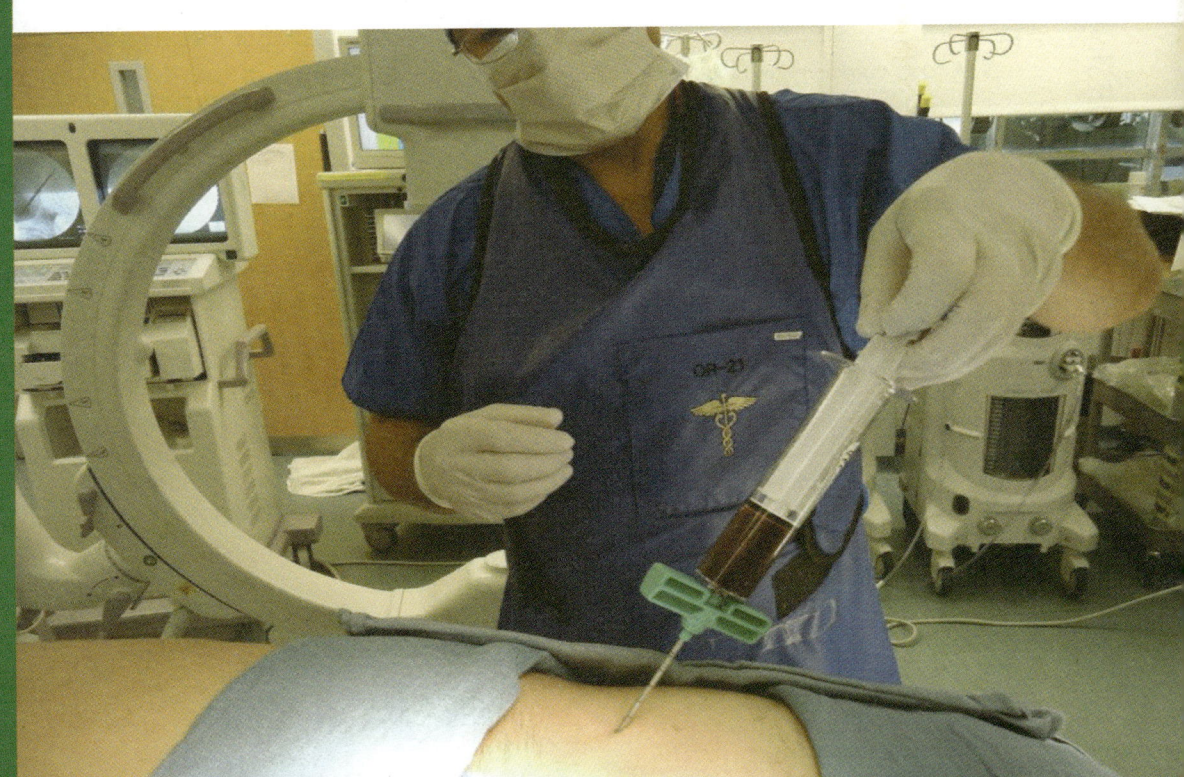

DEFINITION

Assisting in obtaining bone marrow sample which is aspirated from various bone like sternum/ilium/tibia using aseptic technique.

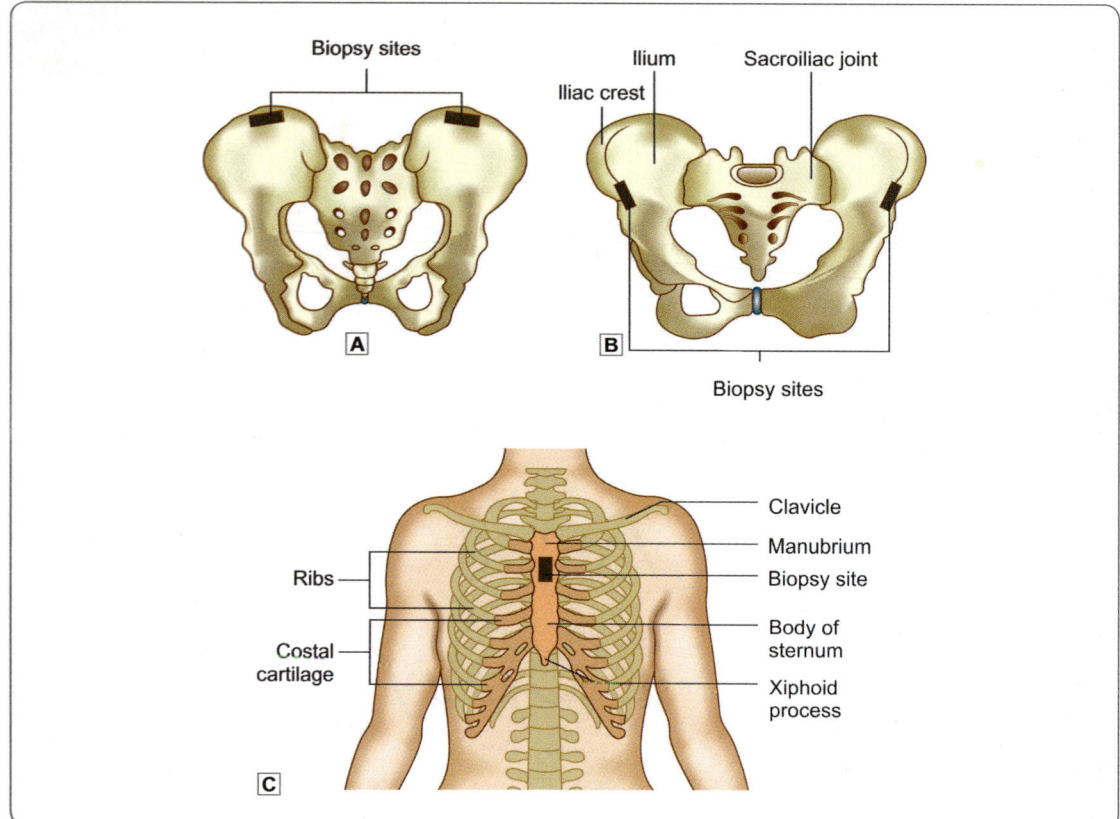

FIGS 1A TO C: Common sites for bone marrow aspiration. **A.** Posterior iliac crests; **B.** Anterior iliac crests; **C.** Sternum

PURPOSES

- ❑ To diagnose hematological disorders
- ❑ To follow the course of disease and patient's response to treatment
- ❑ To diagnose various diseases such as primary metastatic tumor, infectious disease and certain granulomas.
- ❑ To isolate bacteria and other pathogens by culture.

ARTICLES REQUIRED AND THEIR PURPOSES

Articles	Purposes
A clean tray containing:	
❑ 5cc syringe	❑ To collect bone marrow
❑ Needle no 22 & 20	❑ To insert into the bone
❑ Sterile gloves	❑ To avoid cross infection
❑ Lignocaine 2%	❑ To reduce pain

Contd...

Articles	Purposes
❑ Small bottle with formalin, alcohol, acetic acid (FAA)	❑ To collect bone marrow
❑ Culture tubes	❑ To preserve bone marrow
❑ Slides	❑ To observe
❑ Mackintosh and draw sheet	❑ To avoid soiling of the linen
❑ Adhesive tapes and scissors	
❑ Tincture benzoin solution	❑ To reduce infection
❑ Kidney tray	❑ To collect the waste

STEPS OF PROCEDURE AND RATIONALE

Steps	Rationale
❑ Check the physicians order and nursing care plan and investigation reports like coagulation studies	❑ To obtain specific information
❑ Take the concerned from the patient	❑ To fulfil the legal requirement
❑ Explain the procedure to the patient	❑ To relieve anxiety and gain cooperation from the patient
❑ Provide privacy to the patient and shave the site if necessary	❑ To avoid unnecessary exposure of the patient
❑ Provide supine position for sternal puncture and lateral position for iliac crest puncture	
❑ Assist the physician to clean the site with solution and drape with sterile towel	❑ Reduces risk for infection
❑ Explain to the patient that anesthetic drug is to be given	❑ Prepares patient to anticipate what he will be experiencing
❑ Continue to observe and reassure the patient as the physician punctures and aspires the marrow (Fig. 2)	

FIG. 2: Bone marrow aspiration to collect specimen

Steps	Rationale
❑ Aspirate bone marrow in syringe and collect specimen in various containers	❑ Bone marrow tissue is collected in containers with FAA
❑ After the syringe is removed apply pressure over the site for about 5–10 minutes using a sterile swab till the bleeding stops	❑ It minimizes bleeding and hematoma formation
❑ When bleeding stops, seal the puncture site with tincture benzoin and apply firm dressing	❑ To avoid oozing from puncture site

Contd…

Assisting with Bone Marrow Aspiration and Biopsy

Steps	Rationale
❑ Advice the patient not to wash or wet the puncture site for 1 or 2 days	❑ It provides an air tight seal to the puncture site and prevents entry of bacteria
❑ Make the patient comfortable. Instruct the patient that he/she may be mobile after 4–6 hours	❑ To make the patient comfortable
❑ Replace the articles to the utility room	❑ To utilize it for sterilization
❑ Send specimen to laboratory with necessary data in the form and container properly labeled	❑ To avoid mismatch of the sample
❑ Record the procedure in the patient's record	

COMPLICATIONS

❑ Bleeding
❑ Infection

Points to Remember

❑ The site for biopsy for children below 2 years is tibia.
❑ Children needs to be sedated before aspiration.

CHAPTER 38

Assisting with Renal Biopsy

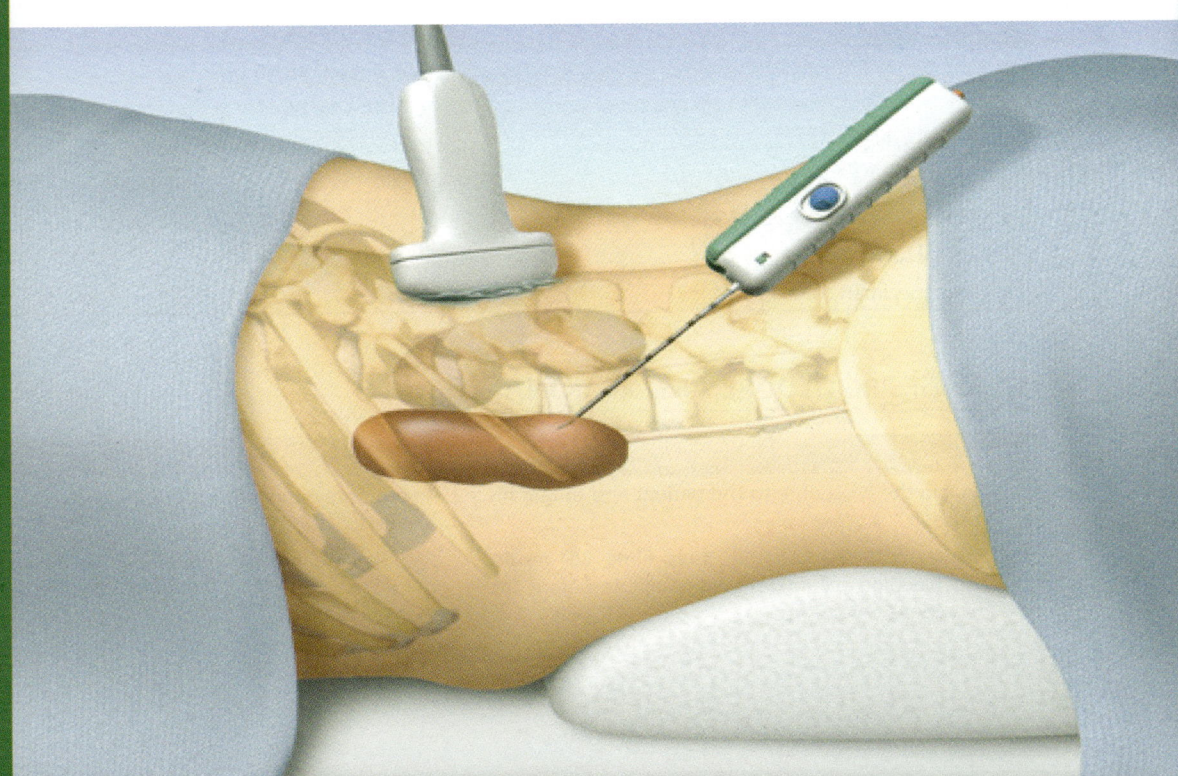

DEFINITION

A renal biopsy is a procedure used to extract kidney tissue for laboratory analysis.

Assisting with insertion of a percutaneous needle under ultrasound guidance to obtain a biopsy specimen from kidney.

PURPOSES

- ❑ To diagnose the cause of glomerulonephritis
- ❑ To diagnose renal malignancy
- ❑ Before renal transplantation
- ❑ To evaluate rejection response in renal transplant patient
- ❑ To determine prognosis of renal disease.

ARTICLES REQUIRED AND THEIR PURPOSES

Articles	Purposes
A sterile tray containing:	
❑ Artery clamp	❑ To clamp the sterile cloth gown
❑ Surgical towels–2	❑ To maintain sterile field
❑ Bowl with cotton swabs	
❑ Kidney tray	❑ To collect the waste
❑ Sterile biopsy needle	❑ To collect the tissue
❑ Scalpel blade 3/11 with holder	❑ To hold the needle
❑ Slit towel	❑ To avoid the soiling
A clean tray containing:	
❑ Iodine, spirit or any antiseptic solution	❑ To clean the site
❑ 2% xylocaine	❑ To reduce localized pain
❑ Sand bag or firm pillow	❑ To maintain proper posture
❑ Adhesive tape	❑ To fix the needle
❑ 10% formalin	❑ To store biopsy material
❑ 5cc syringe	
❑ Disposable needles 22G, 20G	
❑ Normal saline	
❑ Urine specimen container	

STEPS OF PROCEDURE AND RATIONALE

Steps	Rationale
❑ Explain the procedure to the patient and obtain his consent	❑ To promote patient's cooperation and reduces his anxiety
❑ Ensure all the reports like X-ray films, IVP results and bleeding parameters are available before the procedure	❑ Provide baseline data and determine treatment guidelines

Contd...

Steps	Rationale
❑ Assemble all the equipment trolley at the treatment room	❑ Saves time, material and energy
❑ Assist the patient to lie down in a prone position and provide a pillow under the abdomen	❑ Provide access to biopsy site
❑ The site is prepared by cleaning with betadine or savlon	❑ Minimize the risk of introducing microorganism in the body
❑ Assist in making a stab incision through skin and inserting biopsy needle	
❑ Advise the patient to take deep breath while taking biopsy	❑ Avoids chances of injury to adjacent organs
❑ Apply pressure and bandages on the site while removing the needle	❑ Pressure over incision site prevents bleeding
❑ Make the patient to turn in supine position and make him comfortable	
❑ Biopsy specimen should be preserved in formalin solution before sending it to laboratory	
❑ Replace all the articles and document the time of biopsy, vital signs, success of the procedure	

CONTRAINDICATIONS

❑ Single functioning kidney
❑ Malignancy
❑ Hydronephrosis
❑ Coagulation disorders

NOTES

CHAPTER 39

Endoscopy
(Esophagogastroduodenoscopy/ Esophagogastroscopy)

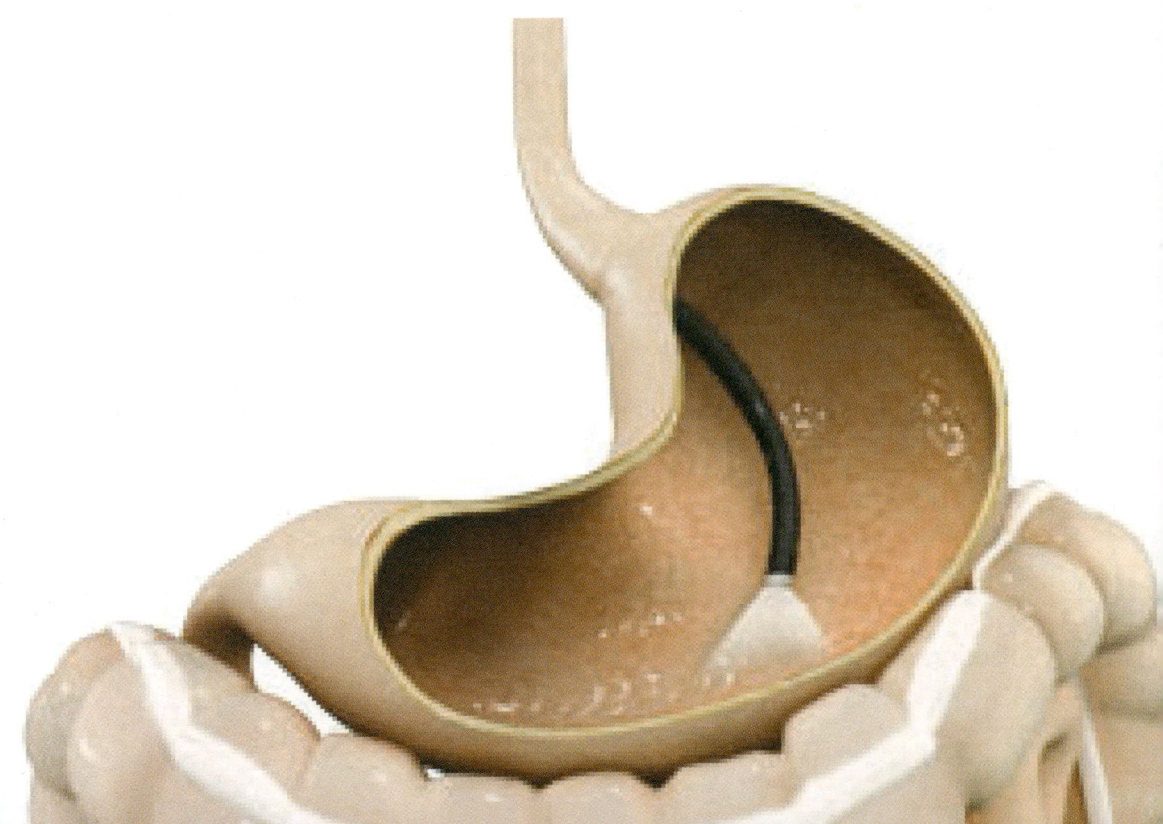

INTRODUCTION

Esophagogastroscopy includes gastroscopy and esophagoscopy. A flexible fiberoptic endoscope is used to direct visualization of internal structure of esophagus, stomach and duodenum. Suction can be applied for removal of foreign bodies. The test performed under local or Intravenous (IV) sedation.

DEFINITION

Endoscopy is a visual examination of esophagus, stomach and first part of small intestine (duodenum) by the use of special instrument called as endoscope.

PURPOSES

- ❑ To visualize gastric mucosa for diagnostic and therapeutic purpose
- ❑ To treat upper GI conditions
- ❑ To obtain specimen

INDICATIONS

- ❑ Esophageal: Esophageal and varices, epigastric pain, gastroesophageal reflux disease (GERD), neoplasms,
- ❑ Esophageal and gastric varices
- ❑ Chronic GI bleeding
- ❑ Strictures
- ❑ Gastric ulcer
- ❑ Neoplasm

CONTRAINDICATIONS

- ❑ Possible perforation
- ❑ Medically unstable patient.
- ❑ Unwilling patient.
- ❑ Anticoagulation, pharyngeal diverticulum
- ❑ Head and neck surgery.

NURSING CONSIDERATIONS

Prior Procedure

- ❑ Explain procedure to the patient and his relatives.
- ❑ Take written consent
- ❑ Instruct the patient to restrict food and fluid for 8–12 hours before the test
- ❑ Remove dentures, eyeglasses and jewelry before test.
- ❑ Instruct the patient to void.
- ❑ Check vital signs of the patient.
- ❑ Provide comfort and remove patients fear, anxiety about the procedure.
- ❑ Patient may take prescribed medication at 6 am on the day of test.
- ❑ Keep ready specimen containers with proper labeling.

During Procedure

- ❑ Sedation may be given prior to the procedure to relax the patient as per doctor's order.

- ❑ The procedure takes approximately 1 hour.
- ❑ Make sure that the dentures, eyeglasses and jewelery are removed.
- ❑ Explain the patient that he/she may feel some pressure and fullness in stomach, intestine areas.
- ❑ Monitor vital signs.

After Care

- ❑ Monitor vital signs of the patient.
- ❑ Check the gag reflexes before offering anything orally by asking the patient to swallow or by touching the posterior pharynx with a cotton ball if the throat was sprayed by an anesthetic agent.
- ❑ Inform patient that he/she may feel flatus/gas, which is normal.
- ❑ Provide analgesics for throat discomfort as ordered.
- ❑ Provide support to the patient and family.
- ❑ Observe patient for any complication.

COMPLICATION

Perforation of gastric mucosa.

Point to Remember

- ❑ Check the gag reflux before offering anything orally after the procedure.

NOTES

CHAPTER 40

Cystoscopy

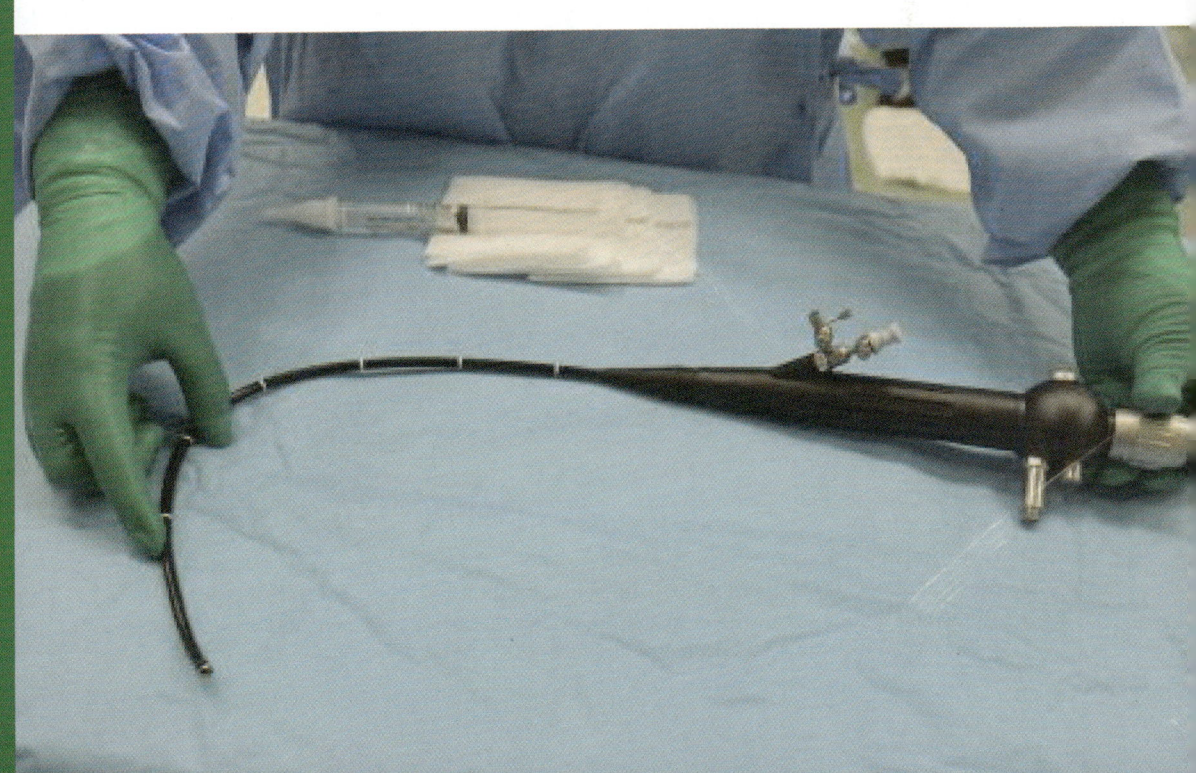

INTRODUCTION

Cystoscopy is the process of viewing a patient's urinary passage and bladder through an instrument introduced through their urinary passage. The instrument is called cystoscope (Fig. 1).

PURPOSES

- ❑ To visualize urinary passage and bladder.
- ❑ To detect various disorder of urinary tract and bladder.

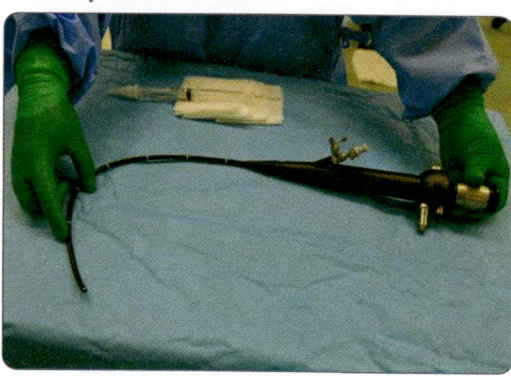

FIG. 1: Cystoscope

INDICATIONS

- ❑ Repeated attacks of urinary tract infection.
- ❑ Hematuria.
- ❑ Involuntary leakage of urine from the urethra (incontinence).
- ❑ Any difficulty in passing urine—either in starting or completing urination, urgency in urination or not being able to empty the bladder fully.
- ❑ Painful urination not responding to conservative management.
- ❑ Enlargement of the prostate.
- ❑ Stones in the urethra or the urinary bladder.
- ❑ Unusual growth in the urinary tract.

NURSING CONSIDERATIONS

Prior Procedure

- ❑ A cystoscopy can be done in an outpatient department or inpatient.
- ❑ Explain the procedure to the patient and his relatives.
- ❑ Take written consent.

During Procedure

- ❑ Give position to the patient (women's to lie on their back with their knees raise and apart, while men to lie down or sit.
- ❑ Give local or general anesthesia as ordered.
- ❑ Clean private part of patient with an antiseptic solution.
- ❑ The doctor gently passes the cystoscope through the urinary passage and a sterile solution (usually normal saline) will flow through the instrument.

- Inform the patient that he/she may feel discomfort and urge to pass urine.
- Mostly, the entire procedure takes about 15–20 minutes.

After Care

- Monitor vital signs regularly for a few hours (every 15–30 minutes).
- Inform patient that the burning sensation while passing urine or blood in urine can occur after an instrumentation. It will be normal within 1 or 2 days after the procedure
- Encourage to take plenty of fluids after the procedure so the bladder and urinary passage gets clear.
- Provide a warm bath or a damp washcloth over the urethral opening to relief any discomfort while urinating.
- Antibiotics might be given for a few days following the procedure to prevent infection.
- In most of the cases, normal food and normal activities can resume after cystoscopy. In some cases, one day observation is required.

NOTES

CHAPTER 41

Proctoscopy

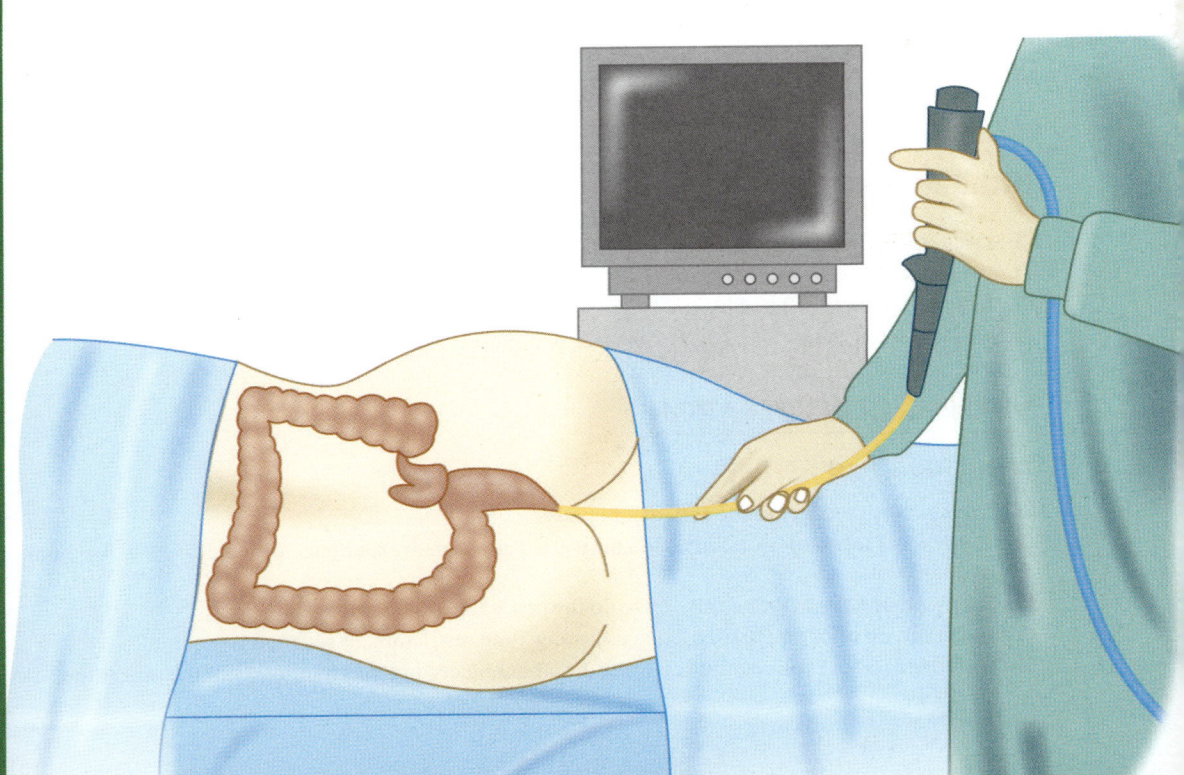

INTRODUCTION

Proctoscopy is a common procedure in which an instrument called proctoscope is used to examine rectal polyps and might be mildly uncomfortable as the proctoscope is inserted further into the rectum (Fig. 1). Modern fiber-optic proctoscopes allow more extensive observation with less discomfort.

DEFINITION

A proctoscopy is visualization of anus, rectum and large intestine. This procedure is also called rigid sigmoidoscopy.

PURPOSES

- ❑ To visualize entire rectal cavity and sigmoid colon.
- ❑ To examine the severity of rectal anal diseases.

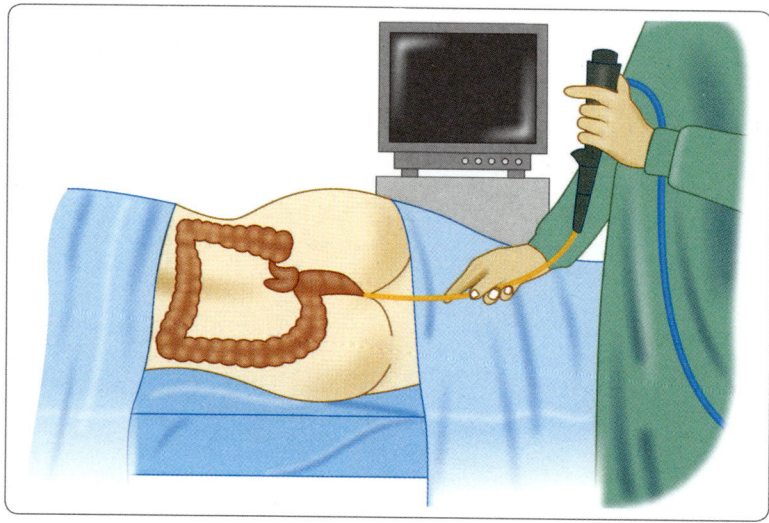

FIG. 1: Proctoscopy

INDICATIONS

- ❑ Diagnose cancer and hemorrhoids
- ❑ Find the cause of bleeding rectum
- ❑ Remove a sample of tissue biopsy
- ❑ Monitor rectal cancer after surgery or other treatments

NURSING CONSIDERATION

Prior Procedure

- ❑ Explain the procedure to the patient and his relatives.
- ❑ The process takes 10–15 minutes to complete. Patient may experience discomfort for a few hours after the treatment.
- ❑ Take written consent for permission to do the procedure.
- ❑ Generally, no prior preparation, such as fasting, fluid restriction, or sedation is required.
- ❑ Instruct to remove your clothing, jewelry, or other objects that may interfere with the procedure.

❑ Provide hospital cloth to wear.

❑ Make sure about sensitivity or allergic to any medications, latex and anesthetic agents (local and general).

❑ Check with history of bleeding disorders or if patient is on any anticoagulant (blood-thinning) medications, aspirin, or other medications that affect blood clotting. It may be necessary for you to stop these medications prior to the procedure as per order.

❑ Patients who have problems with constipation may be given an enema prior to the procedure.

During Procedure

❑ Ask patient to empty bladder and record the amount, flow rate, and voiding pressure during urination.

❑ Provide position to the patient, supine position on the examination table.

❑ A catheter is inserted into the urethra until it reaches the urinary bladder.

❑ One more additional catheter or pressure probe may be inserted into the rectum or vagina to measure pressure in the abdomen. Alternately, adhesive electrodes may be placed on either side of the anal opening to measure muscle function.

❑ A small amount of fluid is to be injected on room temperature through the catheter into the bladder. Ask the patient to describe all sensations, such as warmth, the need to urinate, discomfort or pain, and nausea.

❑ A cytometer is used to measure the bladder pressure by connecting the catheter.

❑ Ask the patient to empty the bladder while the pressure is being recorded when the bladder is completely full,

❑ In some situations, when the patient is on medication that can affect the bladder's muscle tone, the procedure will be repeated in 20–30 minutes.

❑ Remove the catheter once procedure is over.

After Care

❑ Mostly patient can resume usual diet and activities.

❑ Advice the patient to drink extra fluids to dilute the urine and reduce urinary discomfort, such as burning micturition.

❑ Patient may feel some urinary discomfort, but it will reduce over a period of time.

❑ Sitz bath or a tub bath is to be advised as a comfort measure to reduce discomfort.

❑ Inform the patient that he may notice blood in his urine for some time after the procedure. The amount of blood will reduce gradually over the time.

❑ Advice the patient to report doctor immediately if he has complaints about abdominal pain, fever or chills, continued or increased blood in the urine, and if urine output is less than usual amount.

COMPLICATIONS

❑ Urgent need to urinate

❑ Nausea

❑ Sweating

❑ Flushing

❑ Feeling flushed

❑ Headache

❑ High blood pressure

Proctoscopy

NOTES

CHAPTER 42

Endoscopic Retrograde Cholangio-pancreatography

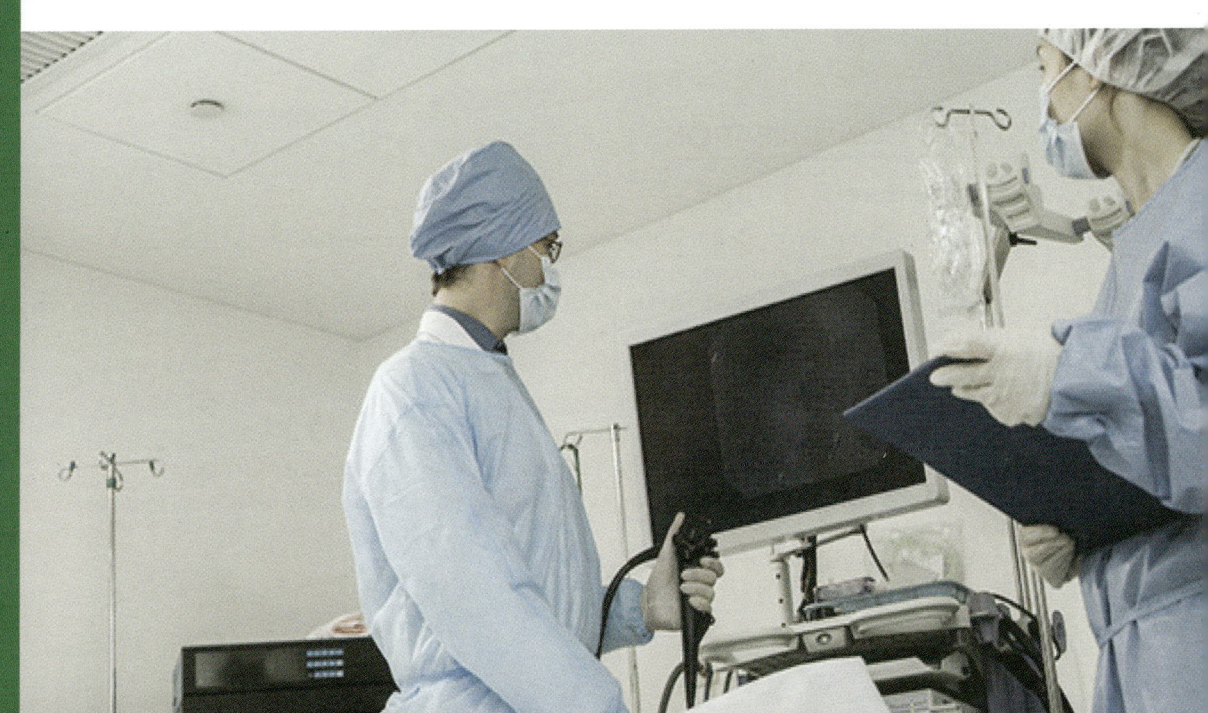

INTRODUCTION

Endoscopic retrograde cholangiopancreatography (ERCP) is a procedure that combines upper gastrointestinal endoscopy and X-ray to treat problems of the bile and pancreatic ducts. ERCP is usually performed under general anesthesia. ERCP uses an endoscope, which is a long flexible narrow tube with a camera at the end. ERCP can provide important information that cannot be obtained by abdominal ultrasound, CT scan or MRI.

DEFINITION

ERCP is a diagnostic procedure done to examine diseases of the liver, bile ducts and pancreas.

PURPOSES

- ❑ To inspect internal organs.
- ❑ To determine causes.
- ❑ To help in confirming diagnosis.
- ❑ To guide for accurate treatment choice.

INDICATIONS

- ❑ Blockage of the bile duct
- ❑ Obstruction of the bile duct (jaundice)
- ❑ Persistent or recurrent upper abdominal pain which cannot be diagnosed by MRI, CT
- ❑ Sphincter of (Oddi dysfunction)
- ❑ Infection
- ❑ Acute pancreatitis
- ❑ Tumor

CONTRAINDICATIONS

- ❑ Abdominal pain of unknown cause
- ❑ Hypersensitivity
- ❑ Acute pancreatitis
- ❑ Cardiac diseases

NURSING CONSIDERATION

Prior Procedure

- ❑ Patient should not eat or drink anything for approximately 8 hours before the examination.
- ❑ Inform your physician about current medications you are taking
- ❑ Inform your physician of any allergies to medications, iodine or shellfish to make the examination comfortable.
- ❑ Patient should not drive or operate machinery until the next day.

During Procedure

- ❑ Insert an intravenous line in patients arm to provide a sedative.
- ❑ Provide a liquid anesthetic to gargle or will spray anesthetic on the back of your throat.
- ❑ Monitor vital signs and keep patient as comfortable as possible. In some cases, patient may receive general anesthesia.
- ❑ Instruct patient to lie on the examination table.
- ❑ The procedure often takes 1–2 hours.

After Care

- ❑ Patient will most often stay at the hospital or outpatient center for 1–2 hours after the procedure so the sedation or anesthesia can wear off.
- ❑ In some cases, you may need to stay overnight in the hospital after ERCP.
- ❑ Patient may feel bloating or nausea for a short-time after the procedure.
- ❑ Patient may have a sore throat for 1–2 days.
- ❑ Patient can take normal diet once swallowing reflux has returned to normal.

COMPLICATIONS

The most common ERCP complication is pancreatitis. Other rare complications are:

- ❑ Heart and lung problems
- ❑ Bleeding (after sphincterotomy)
- ❑ Infection in the bile duct
- ❑ Perforation (a tear in the intestine)

NOTES

CHAPTER 43

Colonoscopy

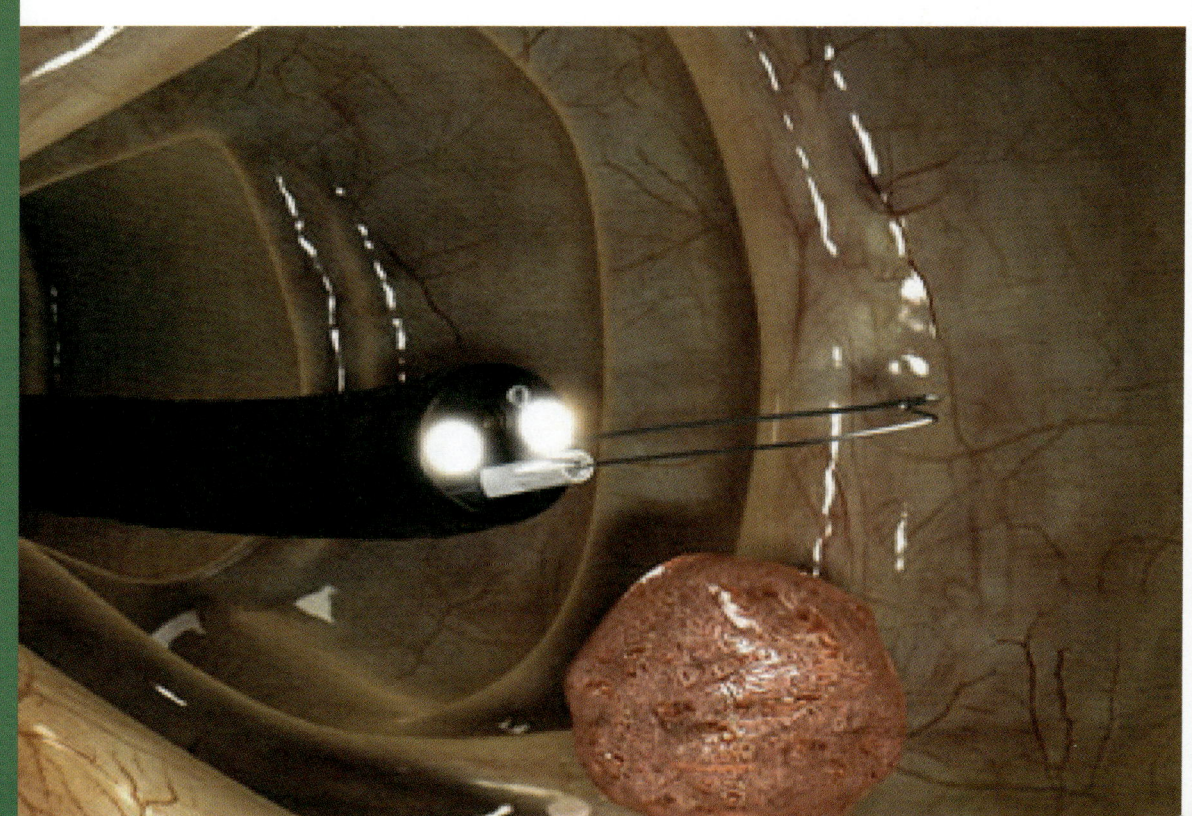

INTRODUCTION

A colonoscopy is an examination used to detect changes or abnormalities in the large intestine (colon) and rectum.

During a colonoscopy, a long, flexible tube (colonoscope) is inserted into the rectum. A tiny video camera at the tip of the tube allows the doctor to view the inside of the entire colon.

PURPOSES

- ❏ To detect colon problems.
- ❏ To reduce your risk of death from colorectal cancer.

INDICATIONS

- ❏ Investigate intestinal signs and symptoms
- ❏ Screen for colorectal cancer
- ❏ Polyps
- ❏ Lower gastrointestinal (GI) bleed
- ❏ Inflammatory bowel disease
- ❏ Acute and chronic diarrhea
- ❏ Therapeutic indications for colonoscopy such as colonic decompression, lower GI bleeding, foreign body removal etc.

CONTRAINDICATIONS

- ❏ Patient's refusal or uncooperative patient
- ❏ Suspected or known case of colonic perforation
- ❏ Severe toxic megacolon
- ❏ Fulminant colitis
- ❏ Recent myocardial infarction

PROCEDURE

Preparation before Procedure

- ❏ Explain procedure to the patient especially about that CO_2 gas will be introduced into colon which may causes discomfort or abdominal cramps.
- ❏ Obtain informed written consent.
- ❏ Keep patient on easily digestible diet 1 week prior colonoscopy to avoid constipation.
- ❏ Ask patient to take low residual diet for 3 days before procedure and nil per oral for 8 hours prior to the colonoscopy.

Bowel Preparation

- ❏ Administer laxative 1–3 days before the procedure.
- ❏ Give cleansing enema in the night before the procedure.
- ❏ Give colonic wash with sodium sulfate or polyethylene glycol dissolved in 5 L of water previous night to the procedure and in the morning of the day of procedure.
- ❏ Administer solution as per doctor's order.
- ❏ Advice patient to take more clear fluids on the day of procedure.

During Procedure

- ❑ Administer sedative if ordered.
- ❑ Provide left lateral position with leg flexed at hip and knee.
- ❑ Instruct patient to take deep breath while tube is inserted.
- ❑ Apply lubricant on the colonoscope and assist in insertion of tube.
- ❑ Apply pressure on areas of abdomen as directed by physician.
- ❑ Monitor vital signs and pain.

AFTER CARE

- ❑ Provide comfort to the patient.
- ❑ Monitor vital signs every 15 minutes in first 1 hour and every 30 minutes for 2 hour.
- ❑ Closely observe for any complication such as bleeding or vomiting.
- ❑ Send well-labeled specimen to the laboratory if required.
- ❑ Record the procedure, time and patient response on nurse's notes.

COMPLICATIONS

- ❑ Infection
- ❑ Perforation
- ❑ Bleeding
- ❑ Hemorrhage

Point to Remember

- ❑ Bowel preparation is most important for colonoscopy.

NOTES

CHAPTER 44

X-ray

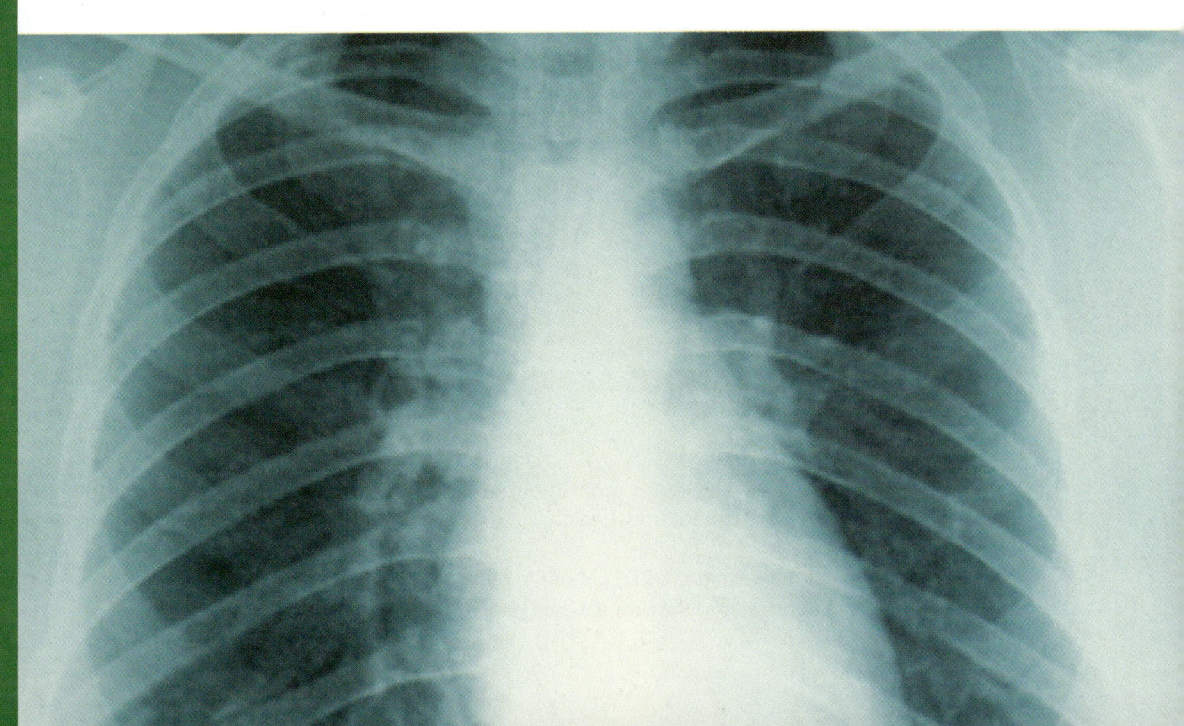

INTRODUCTION

This is a very common diagnostic procedure, which helps in diagnosis of variety of diseases. It is used to examine various organs such as bones, lungs, digestive system, etc.

DEFINITION

X-ray is a radiological examination, which shows various planes and angles of body organ (Fig. 1).

PURPOSES

- ❑ To identify or detect any structural irregularity/abnormality.
- ❑ To rule out disease conditions.
- ❑ To monitor the progress of recovery during illness.
- ❑ To confirm the placement of tube such as Ryle's tube, endotracheal tube.

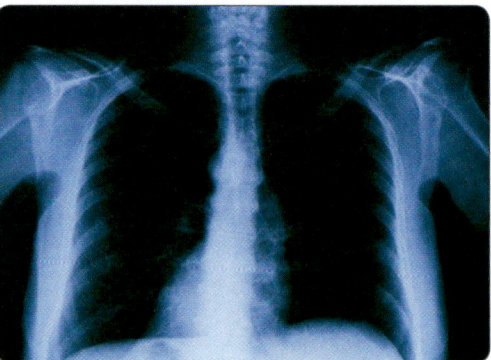

FIG. 1: Chest X-ray

INDICATIONS

- ❑ Injury
- ❑ Diseases
- ❑ When no physical signs and symptoms are present
- ❑ Routine procedure
- ❑ Physical abnormality

CONTRAINDICATION

Pregnancy

NURSING CONSIDERATIONS

Prior Procedure

- ❑ Ask patient to carry case sheet and requisition form. In case of inpatient department (IPD) patients, shift patient to the X-ray department on wheelchair or stretcher as per patient's condition, along with necessary documents.
- ❑ Instruct outpatient department (OPD) patient to report on time.
- ❑ In case of IPD, patients record the timing when patient is been shifted.

During Procedure

- ❑ Hand over patient and documents for X-ray.
- ❑ Provide hospital gown to wear. Assist in changing the gown if require.
- ❑ Ask patient to remove jewelry depending on which body part to be examined.
- ❑ Tell the patient not to do any movements as it leads blurred image.

After Procedure

- ❑ Receive patient in the ward and record arrival timing and X-ray done.
- ❑ Provide comfortable position to the patient.

Point to Remember

- ❑ Inform doctor in case of pregnancy.

NOTES

CHAPTER 45

Ultrasound (Sonography)

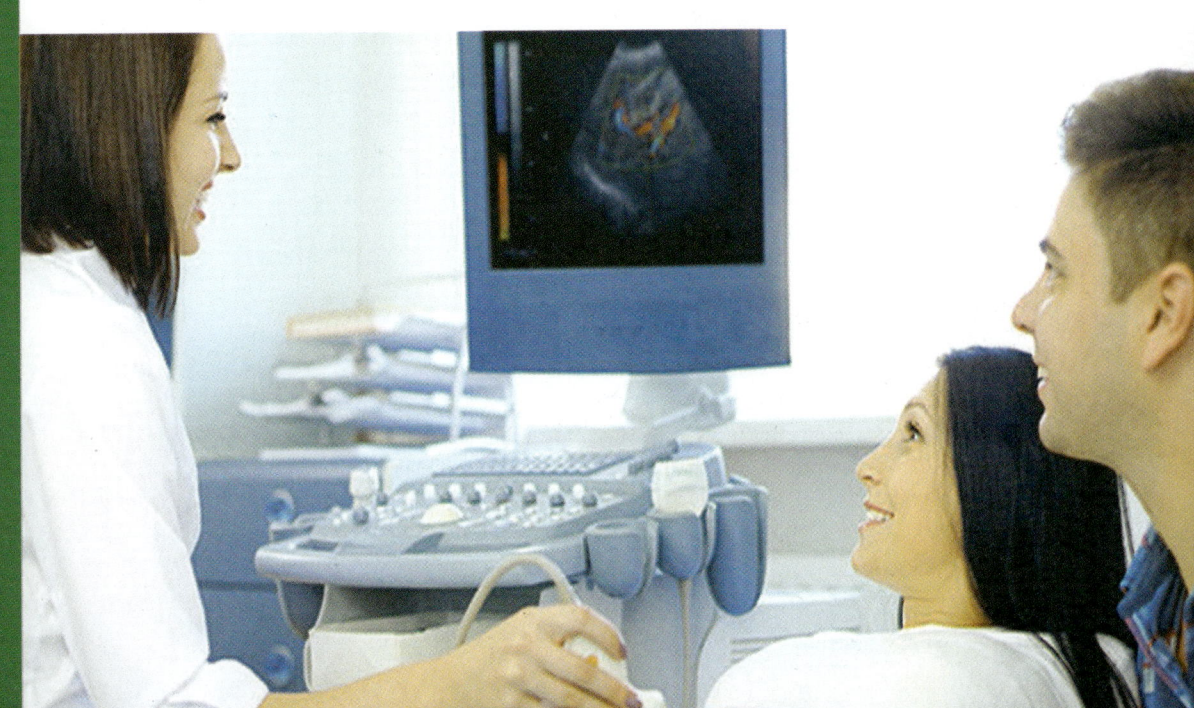

INTRODUCTION

An ultrasound scan is a noninvasive diagnostic imaging technique based on high-frequency sound waves to capture live images soft tissue structure. It is also known as sonography.

DEFINITION

Ultrasonography is a diagnostic medical procedure that uses sound waves to produce images on screen, which allows medical providers to view internal structures of the body.

PURPOSES

- ❑ To confirm accurate diagnosis.
- ❑ To determine gestational age.
- ❑ For investigation of solid organs such as liver, kidney etc.
- ❑ For early detection of various diseases.

Abdominal ultrasound is depicted below in Figure 1.

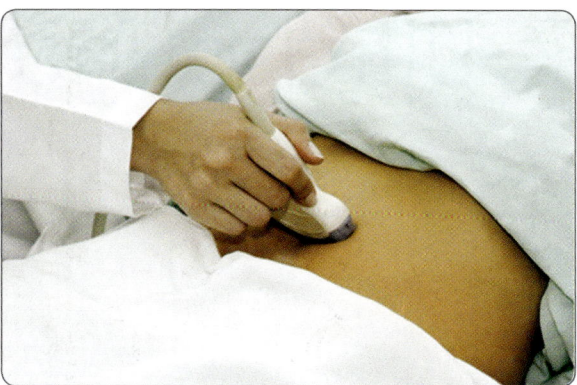

FIG. 1: Abdominal ultrasound

INDICATIONS

- ❑ Routine procedure in pregnancy
- ❑ Pain
- ❑ Swelling
- ❑ Other symptoms that require an internal view of an organ

NURSING CONSIDERATIONS

Prior Procedure

- ❑ Take an appointment.
- ❑ Explain the procedure to the patient. Also inform that the procedure is painless.
- ❑ Report to the department before time with case sheet or prescription sheet.
- ❑ In case of gallbladder, renal artery test, instruct the patient to stop eating and drinking for 8–12 hours before the test.
- ❑ In case of pelvic ultrasounds, ask patient to drink water and not urinate before the test.

During Procedure

- ❑ Provide privacy to the patient and record the started time of the procedure.
- ❑ Apply water-soluble jelly over the skin to be examined.
- ❑ The duration of the exam will vary, but the average is about 30 minutes.

After Care and Documentation

- ❑ Wipe the skin with dry cotton swabs after the procedure.
- ❑ Record the time when the procedure is complete and USG done.
- ❑ Individual can go home immediately and resume normal activities.

NOTES

CHAPTER 46

Electrocardiogram (ECG)

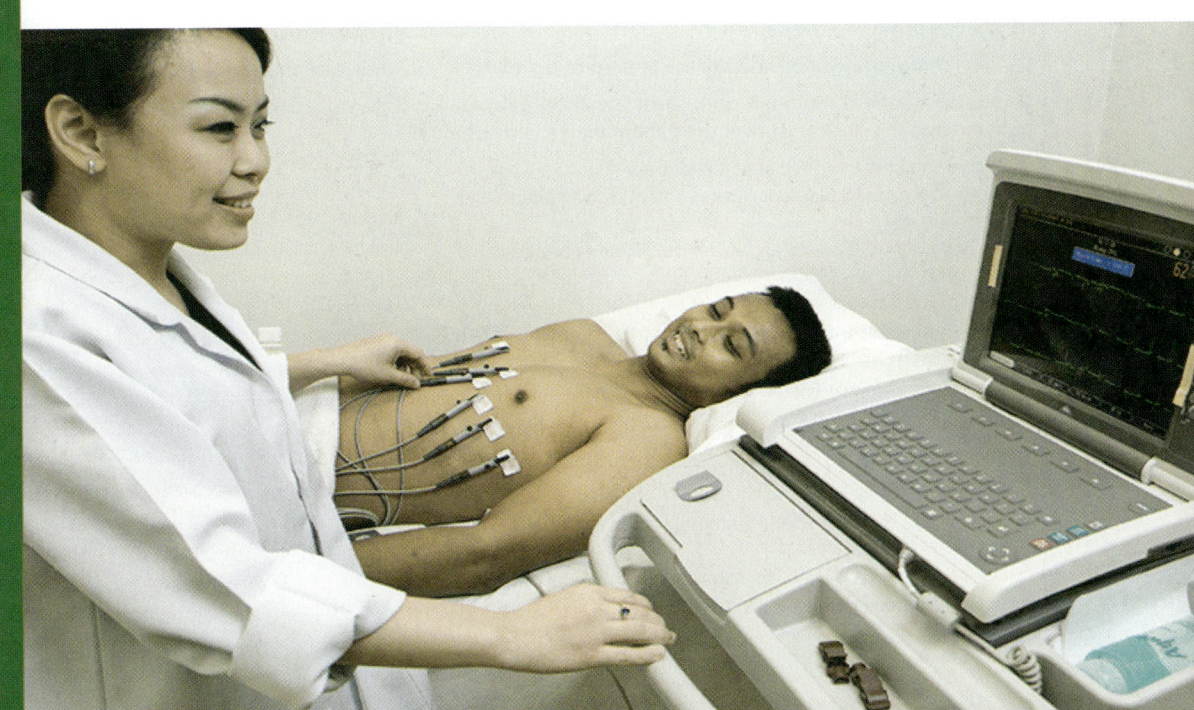

DEFINITION

An electrocardiogram (ECG) records the electrical signal of heart in a graphical form to detect cardiac problems.

PURPOSES

- To assess the cardiac function.
- To diagnose cardiac diseases.
- To assess effect of electrolyte imbalance on cardiac function.
- To evaluate the therapeutic effect.

ARTICLES REQUIRED AND THEIR PURPOSES

Articles	Purposes
❑ ECG machine with 12 lead electrodes	❑ To take an ECG
❑ Electrodes for 12 lead ECG	❑ For electrical recording
❑ Electro conductive gel	❑ For proper conduction between skin and electrodes
❑ Top sheet	❑ To cover patient for comfort
❑ Tissue paper	❑ To wipe the gel

STEPS OF PROCEDURE AND RATIONALE

Steps	Rationale
❑ Ensure proper standardization of ECG machine; set paper speed at 25 mm/minute, provide standard 1 mV signal to ECG machine to receive spikes of 10 mm or 2 large squares in height	❑ For precise recording
❑ Explain the procedure to the patient	❑ To gain cooperation from the patient
❑ Inform that the procedure is safe and painless	❑ To reduce anxiety of the patient
❑ Provide privacy to the patient	❑ To maintain privacy of patient
❑ Provide supine position and ask the patient to be relax	❑ For actual and accurate recording of ECG
❑ Ask the patient to open the chest by loosening or removing the cloth and cover the patient with top sheet	❑ To expose chest area

❑ Shave the chest surface area if required
❑ Apply gel on lead placement sites and attach all electrodes appropriately
  ○ Attach limb leads to all four extremities as per color codes
  ○ Place chest leads appropriately
    ➢ V1 - 4th Intercostal space, just to the right of the sternum
    ➢ V2 - opposite to V1, over the 4th intercostal space at the left sternum border
    ➢ V3 - Midway between V2 and V4
    ➢ V4 - over the 5th intercostal space at the left mid-clavicular line
    ➢ V5 - over the 5th intercostal space at the left anterior axillary line
    ➢ V6 - over the 5th intercostal space at the left midaxillary line	

Contd…

Steps	Rationale

❑ Instruct the patient to remain still in the bed during recording of ECG
❑ Record the ECG
  ○ Automatic recording: Place all leads correctly and ask command for autorecording
  ○ Manual recording: Record limb leads (I, II, III, AVR, AVL, AVF) by setting the machine. Record chest leads (V1–V6) by advancing the suction electrode to the next position after recording each lead	

❑ Check the ECG record for appropriateness	❑ In case of inappropriateness recording needs to be repeated
❑ Remove all electrodes and wipe off the electro conductive gel using tissue paper from the skin and electrodes	❑ After drying the gel may form crust which will interfere in future recording
❑ Label the ECG record with complete detail of patient's identity	❑ Provide patient's identity
❑ Read and report ECG to the physician	❑ To identify any abnormalities

Points to Remember

❑ If the patient needs to be send to the ECG department, always transport patient on trolley.
❑ In case of male patient, shave the chest wall if required for better contact between lead and skin.

NOTES

CHAPTER 47

Electroencephalography (EEG)

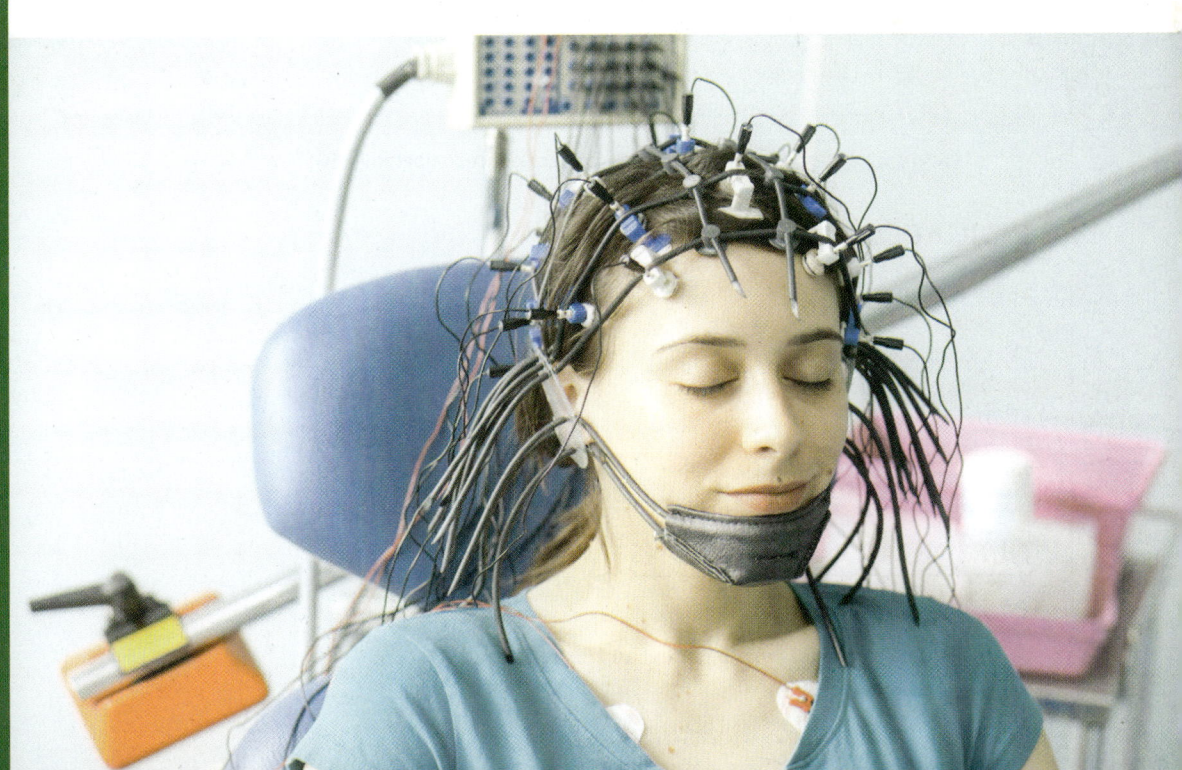

INTRODUCTION

Electroencephalogram (EEG) is a test that detects electrical activity in your brain using small metal discs attached to your scalp. Your brain cells communicate via electrical impulses and are active all the time even when you are asleep.

DEFINITION

Electroencephalography is the recording of an electrical activity by using multiple electrodes (sensors) attached on the scalp of patient and wire connected to the computer.

PURPOSES

- ❑ To rule out various disease conditions of brain.
- ❑ To monitor brain activity during surgery.

Diagram of electroencephalogram (EEG) is depicted below in Figure 1:

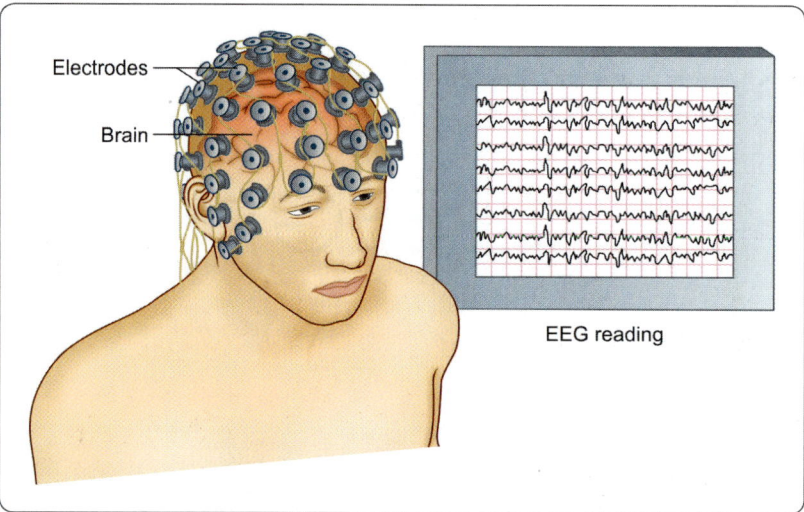

FIG. 1: Electroencephalogram (EEG)

INDICATIONS

- ❑ Brain tumors
- ❑ Seizure
- ❑ Cerebral infarction
- ❑ Intracranial hemorrhage
- ❑ Hematoma
- ❑ Mental disorder
- ❑ Brain infection

NURSING CONSIDERATIONS

Prior Procedure

- ❑ Explain the procedure to the patient and his relatives.

- Instruct to wash hairs the night before the EEG test, and do not apply any products (like sprays or gels) over hairs on the day of the test.
- Avoid eating or drinking anything containing caffeine for at least 8 hours before the test.
- Avoid alcohol 24 hours prior to EEG.
- For adults the recommendation is to sleep not more than 4–5 hours the night prior to the study.
- Take regular medications.

During Procedure

- Provide safety and comfort to the patient.
- Follow instructions given by doctor.

AFTER CARE and Documentation

- Record the date, time and patient's response in nurse's notes.
- Observe for any complication.
- Advise plenty of fluids to rehydrate the patient.

COMPLICATIONS

- Anaphylactic shock
- Cardiac arrhythmias
- Renal failure

Points to Remember

- Wash hairs the night before EEG procedure.
- Avoid caffeine products at least 8 hours before procedure.

Electroencephalography (EEG)

NOTES

CHAPTER 48

Stress Test

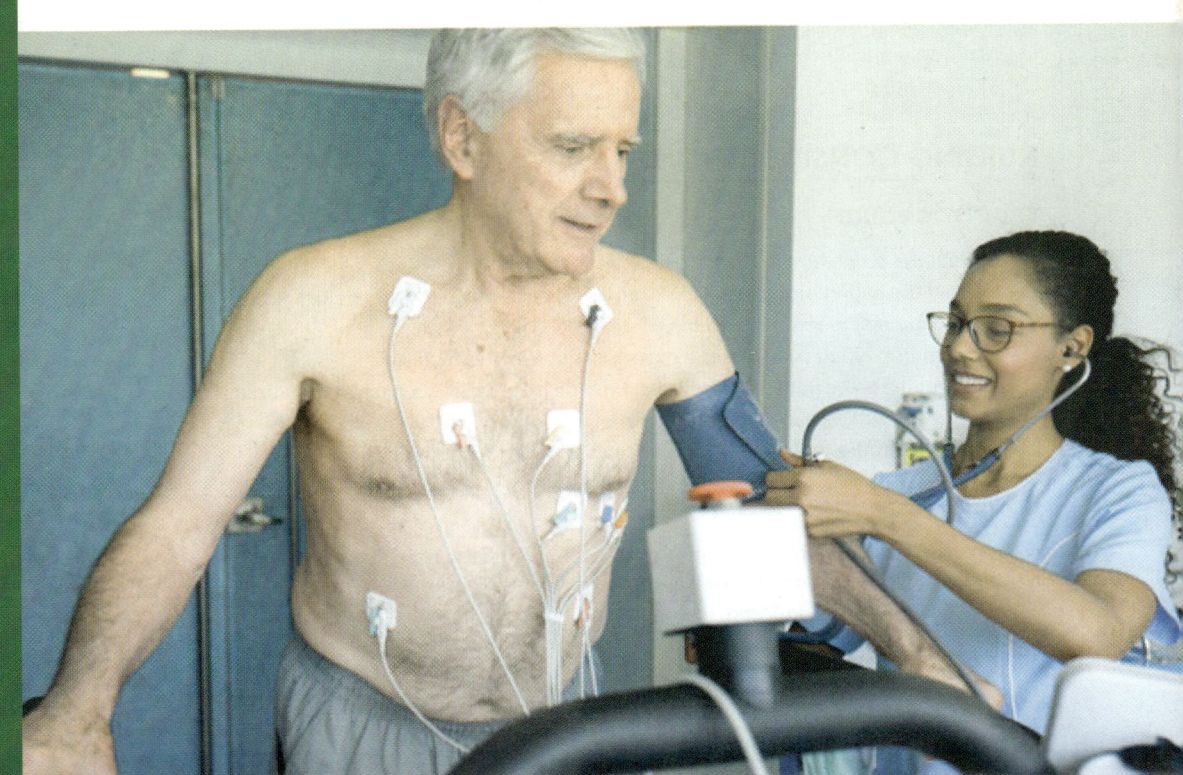

INTRODUCTION

Stress test is a noninvasive procedure to evaluate cardiovascular status of patient who is suffering from cardiac disease or at risk. This test increases the cardiac activity by increasing physical activity.

DEFINITION

Stress test is a method to evaluate cardiovascular response to the physical stress.

PURPOSES

- ❑ To assess cardiac ability (function).
- ❑ To rule out various cardiac disease conditions.
- ❑ To assess people at risk.
- ❑ To evaluate effectiveness of therapeutic treatment.

INDICATIONS

- ❑ Coronary artery disease
- ❑ Risk of coronary artery disease
- ❑ Patient on digoxin therapy
- ❑ Exercise induced arrhythmias

CONTRAINDICATIONS

- ❑ Acute myocardial infarction
- ❑ Uncontrolled systemic hypertension
- ❑ Recent pulmonary embolism
- ❑ Untreated arrhythmias
- ❑ Second and third degree AV block
- ❑ Acute systemic illness
- ❑ Moderate to severe mitral or aortic valve stenosis

NURSING CONSIDERATIONS

Prior Procedure

- ❑ Explain the procedure to the patient and his relatives.
- ❑ Instruct the patient not to eat, smoke and drink alcohol 3–4 hours before test.
- ❑ Instruct patient to remove jewelry.
- ❑ Assess pulse, blood pressure and oxygen saturation before test.
- ❑ Ask to undress the patient up to waist. Provide hospital gown or shirt to patient.
- ❑ Prepare the site with alcohol swabs. If the skin is hairy, shave the site.
- ❑ Attach electrodes to the chest and connect to the stress test machine.

During Procedure

A stress echocardioagram is a test done to assess how well the heart works under stress. The stress can be triggered by either exercise on a treadmill or a medicine called dobutamine.

- ❑ Provide safety and comfort to the patient.

- During a nuclear stress test the individual will exercise, a radioactive dye is injected and then images are taken to assess the heart health.
- Keep emergency drugs and equipment's ready nearby.

After Care and Documentation

- Record the date, time and patient's response in nurse's notes.
- Monitor for complications.
- Advise plenty of fluids to rehydrate the patient.

COMPLICATIONS

- Anaphylactic shock
- Cardiac arrhythmias
- Renal failure

Point to Remember

- Ask patient not to eat, smoke or drink 3-4 hours prior the procedure.

NOTES

CHAPTER 49

Computed Tomography (CT)

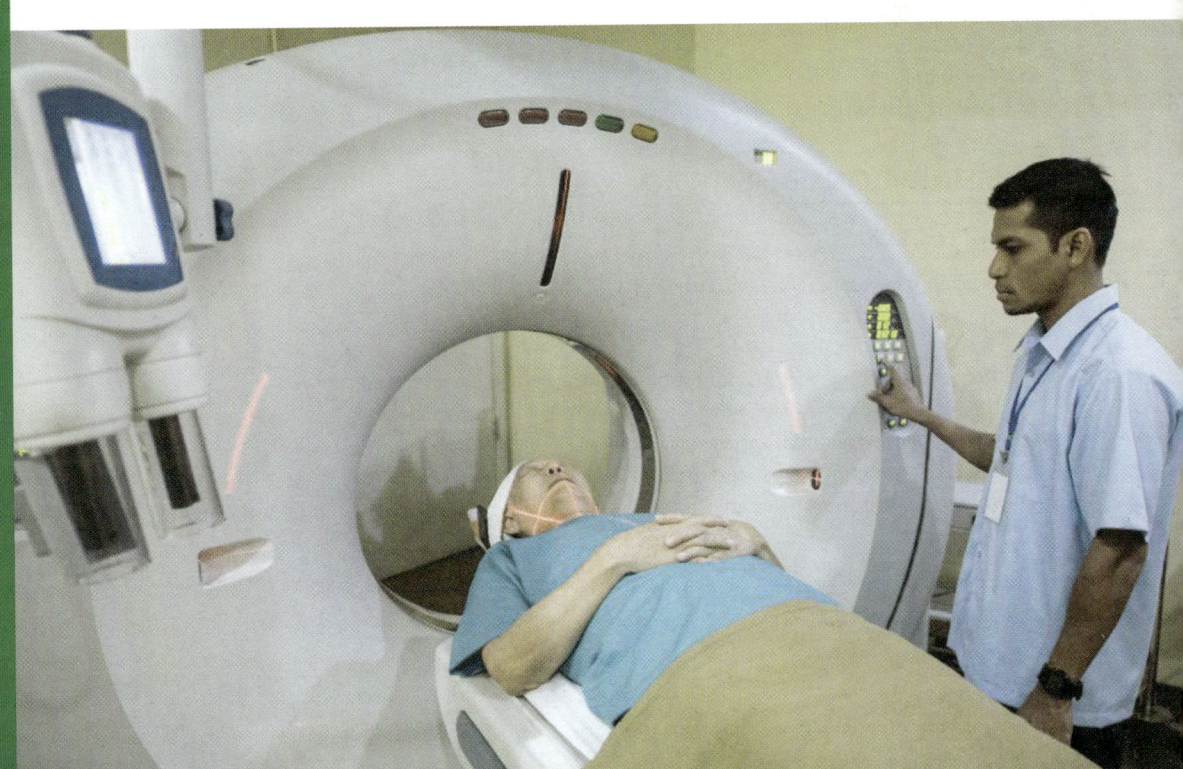

INTRODUCTION

Computed tomography (CT) is an imaging procedure in which X-ray is used to create detailed scans of areas inside the body. It is also called computerized axial tomography (CAT). Computerized tomography scan is 100 times more sensitive than the normal X-ray. In this procedure, radiopaque dye is use to provide contrast scan.

DEFINITION

Computerized tomography is a computerized X-ray that produces detailed images of structures of the body.

PURPOSES

- ❑ It provides information about pathological condition.
- ❑ To make and confirm diagnosis.
- ❑ It shows detailed image of an organ.
- ❑ To detect neoplasm.

INDICATIONS

- ❑ Brain and spinal diseases
- ❑ Bone lesions
- ❑ Hemorrhage
- ❑ Tumors
- ❑ Small delicate structures e.g. ears, sinuses, brain.
- ❑ Post-traumatic patients
- ❑ Cases where MRI is contraindicated

CONTRAINDICATIONS

- ❑ Contrast allergy
- ❑ Renal failure
- ❑ Pregnancy
- ❑ Claustrophobia

NURSING CONSIDERATIONS

Prior Procedure

- ❑ Explain procedure to the patient.
- ❑ Obtain written consent.
- ❑ Take an appointment.
- ❑ Report to the registration counter before time on the day of examination.
- ❑ Please notify doctor if you have any allergy to iodine or contrast.
- ❑ No dietary restriction if contrast is not used.
- ❑ Instruct patient not to eat and drink at least for 4 hours.
- ❑ Adult's or children's who are not cooperative or restless, CT scan can be done under mild sedation/general anesthesia
- ❑ Provide hospital gown to wear.
- ❑ Instruct to remove all jewelry and metal objects from the body.
- ❑ In case contrast scan, skin test is required to check allergic reaction.

- For diabetic patients: If you are taking glucovance, glucophage or metformin (generic), you will need to stop taking these medicines on the day of your examination and up to a minimum of 48 hours after the examination.
- Take any prescribed medications on the day of your test unless instructed not to do so.

During Procedure

- Make the patient comfortable on the table.
- Provide appropriate position depending upon body part.
- Instruct the patient not to move during procedure.
- Assist while administration of contrast.
- Observe for any side effects such as palpitation, itching, restless.
- The procedure lasts for 30–45 minutes.

After Care and Documentation

- If the patient received a contrast injection, remove intravenous (IV) cannula from the arm before going home.
- Encourage more fluid to avoid dehydration.
- In case of sedation received by patient, send the patient home when he/she is fully awake and alert.
- Record the time, duration, tolerance and body part in nurse's notes.

Point to Remember

- Check sensitivity with contrast agent.

NOTES

CHAPTER 50

Magnetic Resonance Imaging (MRI)

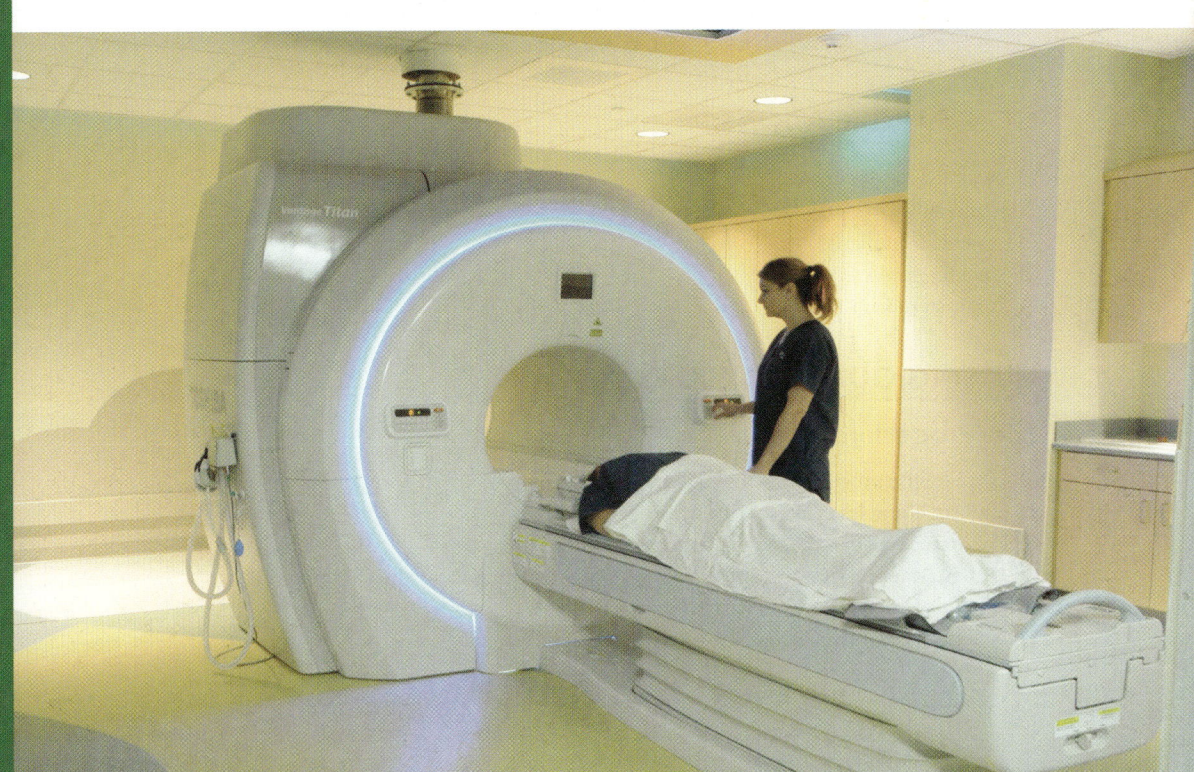

INTRODUCTION

Magnetic resonance imaging (MRI) scan is a noninvasive imaging test that uses powerful magnetic field to obtain images of different body parts in detail. MRI (Fig. 1) also known as nuclear magnetic resonance (NMR) imaging.

DEFINITION

Magnetic resonance imaging technique provides visualization of internal organs through magnetic field and radio frequency waves.

PURPOSES

- ❑ To visualize internal organs and tissues.
- ❑ To detect various pathological conditions.
- ❑ To rule out stages of malignancy.

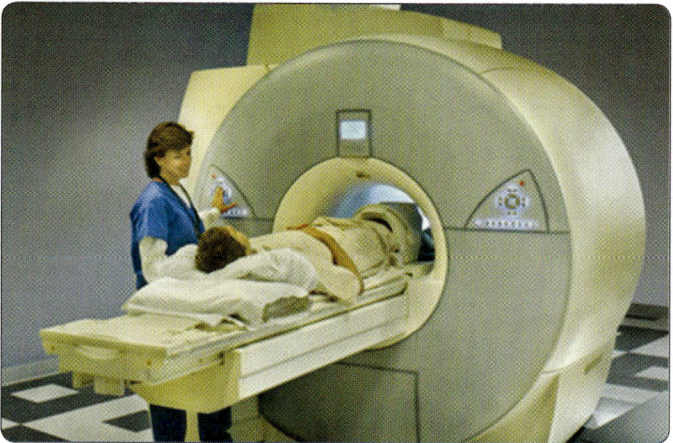

FIG. 1: Magnetic resonance imaging (MRI)

CONTRAINDICATIONS

Electronic devices such as:
- ❑ Pacemaker
- ❑ Cochlear implant
- ❑ Insulin pump
- ❑ Brainstem stimulator

NURSING CONSIDERATIONS

Prior Procedure

- ❑ Explain the procedure to the patient and his relatives.
- ❑ Inform about lot of noises during procedure.
- ❑ Written consent to be taken from the patient.
- ❑ Patient does not require any dietary preparation unless anesthesia is planned.
- ❑ Provide hospital gown to wear.
- ❑ Instruct to remove all jewelry, pins or any metal objects.

During Procedure

- ❑ Tell the patient to empty the bladder before the procedure.
- ❑ Patient will be asked to remain perfectly still during the time the imaging takes place, but between sequences some minor movement may be allowed.
- ❑ Monitor vital signs if indicated.
- ❑ Some patients may require continuous monitoring and support during MRI procedures such as physically or mentally unstable, high-risk cases.
- ❑ Observe for any allergic reactions to contrast medium.

After Care and Documentation

- ❑ Ask the patient to sit first and then stand slowly after the procedure.
- ❑ Evaluate patient's condition.
- ❑ Record the date, duration and patient's response in nurse's notes.

COMPLICATION

Allergy to contrast medium.

Points to Remember

- ❑ Instruct the patient regarding loud noise inside the MRI room.
- ❑ Ask patient to empty the bladder before procedure.

NOTES

CHAPTER 51

Barium Studies

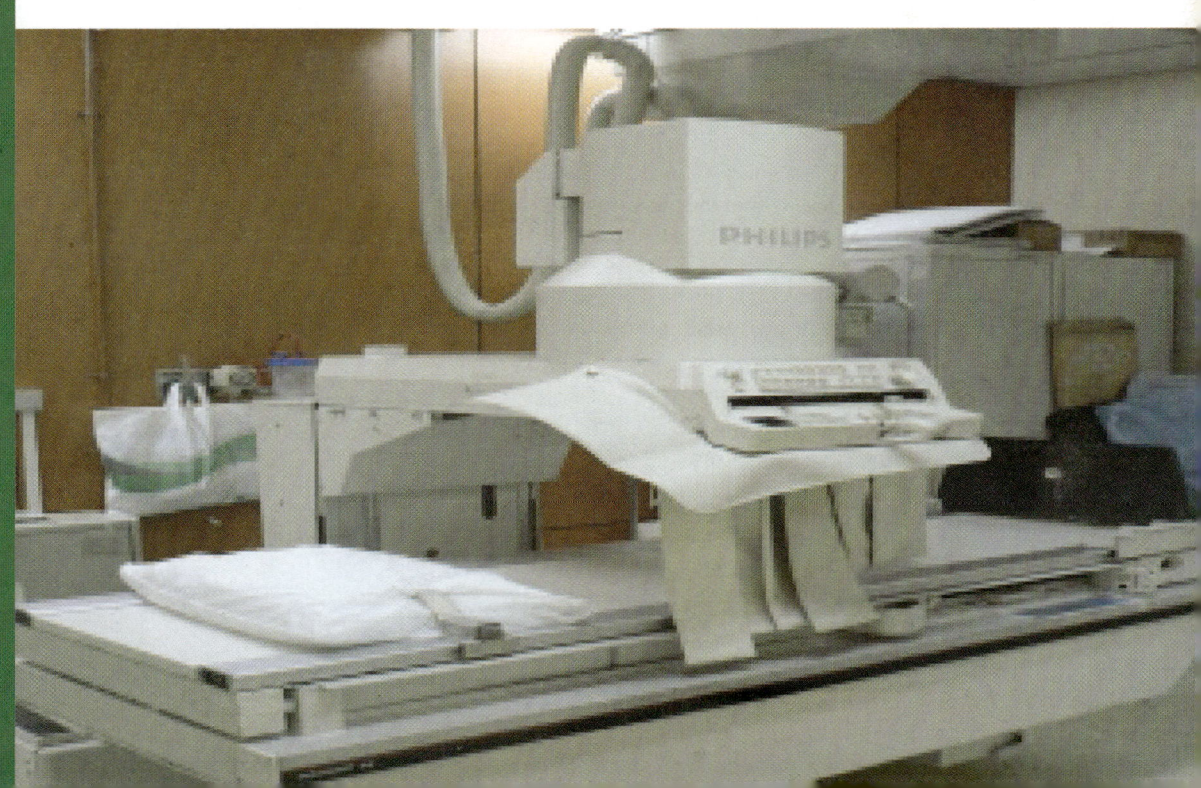

INTRODUCTION

Radiopaque liquid or barium sulfate is introduced as contrast medium into the gastrointestinal tract for proper visualization and taking X-ray. Barium sulfate is odorless, tasteless and completely insoluble powder. It is ingested in the form of aqueous suspension.

DEFINITION

- **Barium swallow:** Barium sulfate suspension is orally administered for radiographic examination of hypopharynx and oropharynx.
- **Barium meal:** Barium sulfate suspension is orally administered for radiographic examination of the upper gastrointestinal tract.

PURPOSES

- To outline the esophagus, stomach, jejunum and ileum.
- To detect abnormalities of esophagus.
- To determine neoplasm.

INDICATIONS

- Esophageal disorder
- Neoplasm
- Abnormalities
- Cyst

CONTRAINDICATIONS

- Gastrointestinal-perforation
- After gastrointestinal (GI) surgery
- Acute illness

NURSING CONSIDERATIONS

Prior Procedure

- Explain about the procedure to the patient and his relatives.
- Take informed consent from the patient and his relatives.
- Instruct to take less residual the diet for 3 days before the procedure and nothing by mouth from midnight prior to test.
- Instruct to avoid smoking in the morning before test.
- Administer premedication as prescribed.

During Procedure

- Provide comfort to the patient.
- Instruct patient that a series of X-ray will be taken.

After Care

- Offer a mouthwash after series of X-ray is completed.
- Provide meal after the completion of the procedure.
- Instruct the patient to increase the fluid intake.
- Mild laxative can be given as ordered.

CHAPTER 52

Barium Enema

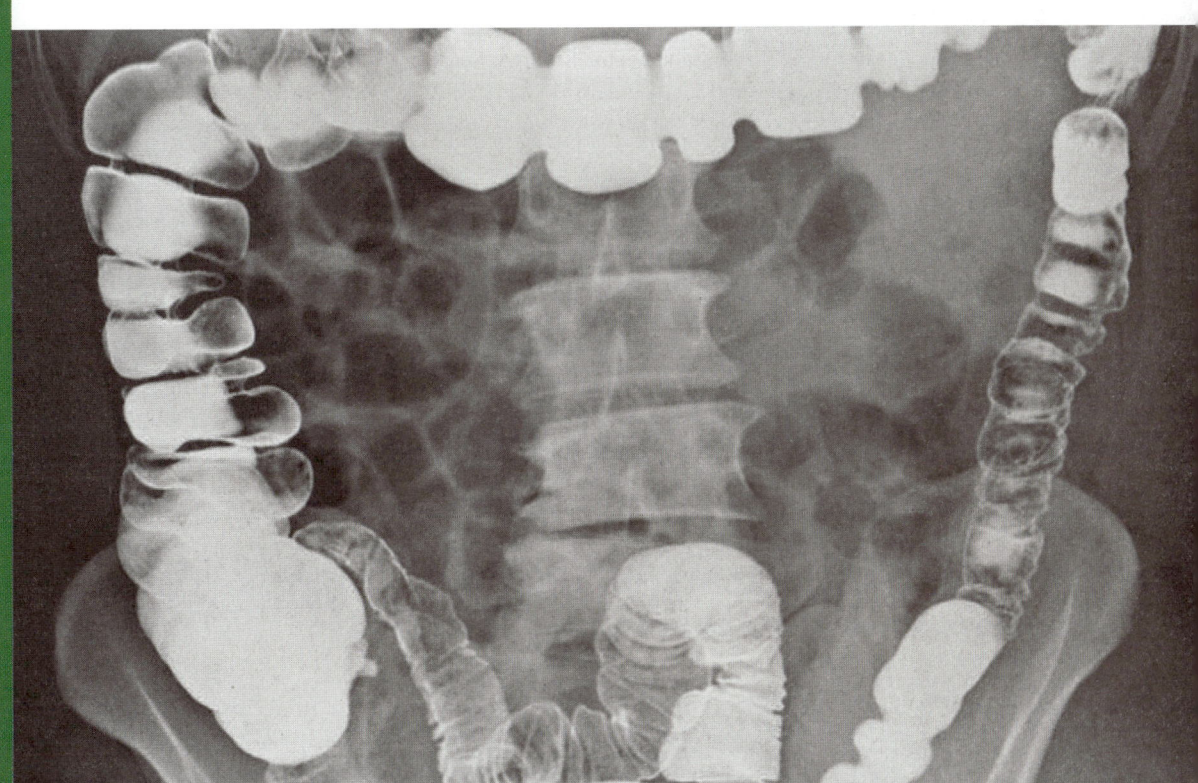

INTRODUCTION

Barium enema is a diagnostic procedure in which radiopaque substance is to be instilled into rectum in order to view large intestine by the fluoroscope. In case of double contrast, gas (CO_2) will be introduced through a tube to distend the large intestine before radiography.

PURPOSES

- ❑ To diagnose diseases of large intestine.
- ❑ To detect neoplasm defects of large intestine.
- ❑ To determine the proper function of large intestine

INDICATIONS

- ❑ Tumor
- ❑ Polyp
- ❑ Ulceration
- ❑ Lesions

CONTRAINDICATIONS

- ❑ Postgastrointestinal surgery
- ❑ Acutely ill patient
- ❑ Allergies

NURSING CONSIDERATIONS

Prior Procedure

- ❑ Explain the procedure to the patient.
- ❑ Instruct the patient about residual diet for 4–5 days preceding the test.
- ❑ Instruct fluid diet on the day before and no food and fluids from midnight.
- ❑ Administer cleansing enema in the previous night and in the morning on the day of procedure is going to be performed.

During Procedure

- ❑ Explain the importance of retaining enema and in different positions.
- ❑ Instill enema fluid as prescribed through rectal tube and the entire colon will be outlined.
- ❑ The procedure takes about 15 minutes.
- ❑ Once the films are taken then expel the enema.

After Care

- ❑ After the procedure, encourage fluid intake.
- ❑ A cleansing enema is given after the test to empty the large bowel.
- ❑ Inform the patient that he/she will pass white colored stools for about 72 hours after procedure due to barium sulfate remaining in the gastrointestinal (GI) tract after procedure.
- ❑ Instruct the patient to report any pain, bloating, absence of stool, bleeding.

Point to Remember

- ❑ Encourage more fluid intake to flush out barium from body.

CHAPTER 53

Intravenous Pyelography (IVP)

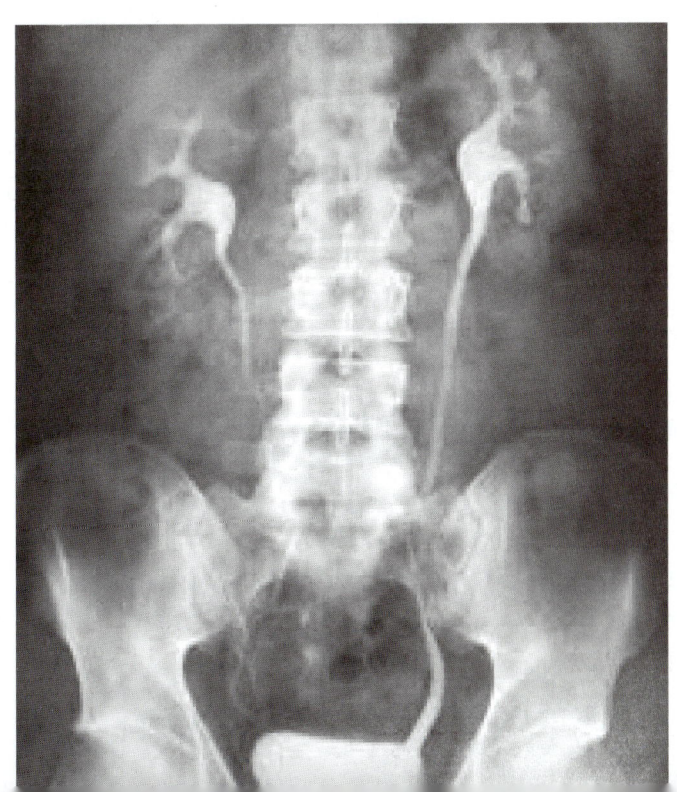

INTRODUCTION

Intravenous pyelography is the visualization of excretory system to determine any structural and pathological changes. It is also called (IVP) excretory pyelogram.

DEFINITION

IVP is the roentgenographic view of kidneys, ureters and bladder by injecting dye into vascular system.

PURPOSES

- ❑ To identify and determine structural changes and blood flow to kidneys, bladder and ureters.
- ❑ To assess renal functions.
- ❑ To rule out congenital anomalies.
- ❑ To detect various conditions, e.g. kidney diseases, infections, stones, injury, tumors, prostate infection.

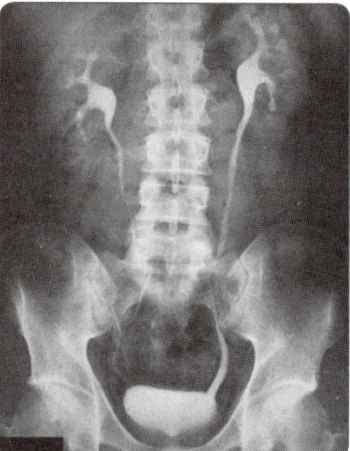

FIG. 1: Intravenous pyelography

INDICATIONS

- ❑ Kidney diseases
- ❑ Kidney infection
- ❑ Injury, tumors, etc.

CONTRAINDICATIONS

- ❑ Hypersensitivity to contrast medium
- ❑ Uncontrolled diabetes
- ❑ Congestive cardiac failure
- ❑ Renal failure

NURSING CONSIDERATIONS

Prior Procedure

- ❑ Explain the procedure to the patient and his relatives.

- ❑ Obtain written consent.
- ❑ Advise to drink lots of fluid the day before and after test, which will help to excrete dye from kidney.
- ❑ Assess for any allergies, especially to iodine or seafood.
- ❑ If patient is taking metformin then stop it 48 hours before and after the procedure after consultation.
- ❑ Ask the patient to stop eating and drinking for12 hours before examination.
- ❑ Ensure that bladder and bowel are empty.
- ❑ Provide supine position to the patient on X-ray table.

During Procedure

- ❑ Provide safety and comfort to the patient.
- ❑ Explain to the patient that there may be feeling of warmth, flushing and salty taste in mouth while injecting dye.
- ❑ Keep emergency drugs and equipments ready nearby.

After Care and Documentation

- ❑ Record the date, time and patient's response in nurse's notes.
- ❑ Observe monitor for complications.
- ❑ Advise plenty of fluids to rehydrate the patient.

COMPLICATIONS

- ❑ Anaphylactic shock
- ❑ Cardiac arrhythmias
- ❑ Renal failure

Intravenous Pyelography (IVP)

NOTES

CHAPTER 54

Preparation and After Care for Mammography

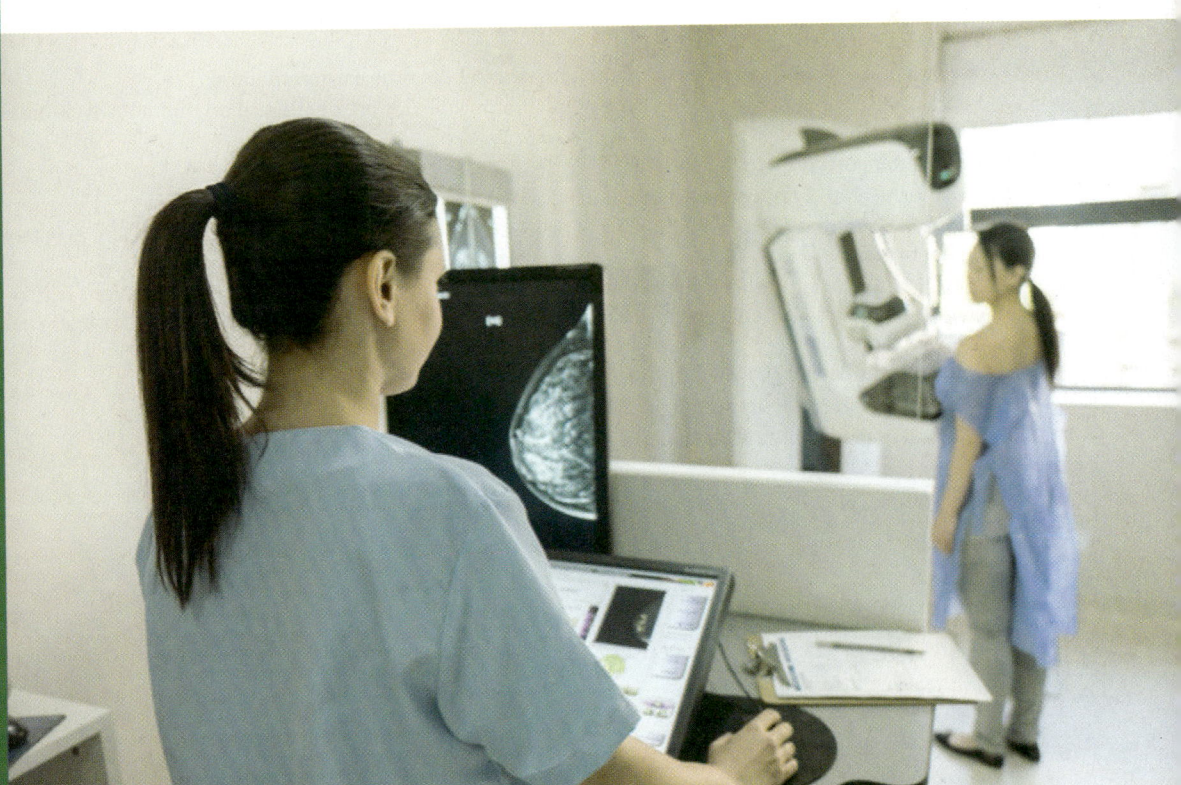

DEFINITION

Mammography is an imaging study which uses low-dose X-ray to examine breasts. It is done to diagnose breast diseases in the women.

COMPUTER AIDED DETECTION (CAD)

CAD is a method that uses a digitalized mammographic image. The computer software then searches for abnormal areas of density calcification or mass which may indicate the presence of cancer. This system highlights the areas on the images which helps in better understanding.

FULL-FIELD DIGITAL MAMMOGRAPHY (FFDM)

In this method, X-ray film is replaced by solid detectors that convert X-rays into electrical signals. The electrical signals are used to produce images of the breast that can be seen on computer or printed on special film.

PURPOSE

To detect early breast cancer in the women with or without symptoms.

CONTRAINDICATION

Pregnancy

STEPS OF PROCEDURE

Preparation of the Patient

- Inform the patient that the best time for a mammogram is 1 week following menstruation.
- Take prior consent from the patient.
- Ask patient to bring along prior mammogram if any at the time of examination.
- Instruct the patient not to use any type of talcum powder, lotion, deodorant on under arms or breasts on the day of examination.
- Explain the procedure to the patient.
- Provide hospital clothing to the patient to wear. Ask to remove jewelry and brassier.
- Inform patient that position of breast will be given by technologist inside the unit and she may feel pressure on her breast
- Inform patient that the technologist will stand behind a glass shield during X-ray. Patient will be asked to change the positions between the images and must hold very still and hold breathing for few seconds while X-ray is taken.
- This procedure may take 30 minutes.
- Ask and help the patient to change the hospital clothing.
- Tell patient that when will she receive report.

CHAPTER **55**

Initial Care of Patient
in the Burn Unit

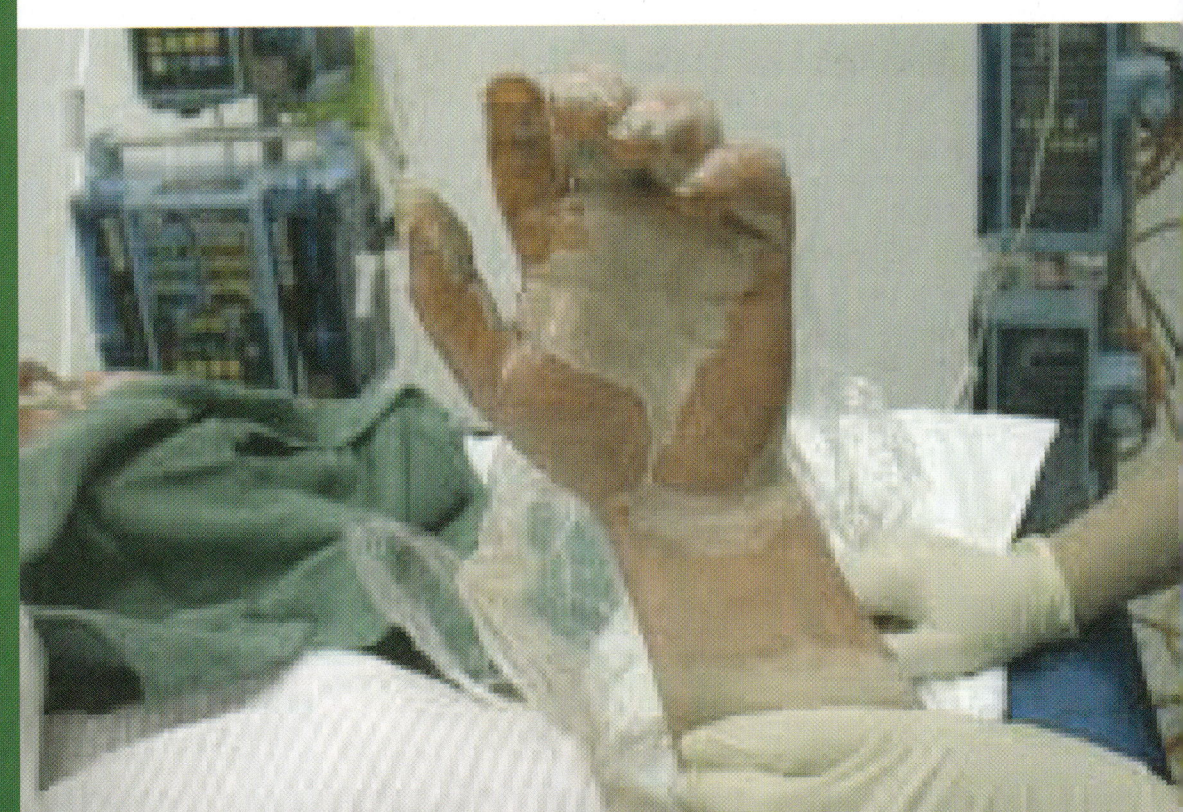

DEFINITION

Admit and initiate care for the burn patient in burn unit.

PURPOSES

- ❑ To save life of the patient
- ❑ To provide fluid resuscitation
- ❑ To relief pain and discomfort
- ❑ To prevent infection
- ❑ To provide wound care

ARTICLES REQUIRED AND THEIR PURPOSES

Articles	Purposes
❑ Sterile bed linen	❑ To provide sterile field
❑ Personal protective equipments (PPE)	❑ To prevent cross infection
❑ Sterile syringes and investigation tubes	❑ To withdraw blood sample
Articles for:	
❑ Intravenous infusion	❑ For fluid replacement
❑ Urinary catheterization	❑ To maintain intake output
❑ Monitor vital signs	❑ To monitor vital organs
❑ Electrocardiogram (ECG) monitoring	❑ To detect cardiac arrhythmias
❑ Nasogastric tube intubation	❑ To provide nutrients

STEPS OF PROCEDURE AND RATIONALE

Steps	Rationale
❑ Prepare unit before receiving patient. Avoid air conditioned room as far as possible at least for 48 hours to prevent complications like hypothermia and compartment syndrome.	❑ To avoid inconvenience and delay in treatment
❑ Assess airway, breathing and circulation	❑ For better management
❑ Provide oxygen as per order	❑ For tissue survival
❑ Check vital signs	❑ To monitor vital organs
❑ Provide immediate care	❑ To promote comfort and prevent infection
❑ Irrigate chemical burn	❑ To remove toxins from the skin surface area
Remove jewelry and clothing	❑ To prevent infection
❑ Collect data about the incident such as cause of burns, time of incident from patient or relatives	❑ It helps in treatment plan
❑ Do complete assessment of patient for location, size, depth and any other trauma	❑ To provide adequate care

Contd…

Steps	Rationale

❏ Assess percentage of burns by rule of 9
   ○ Head and neck–9%
   ○ Anterior thorax–18%
   ○ Posterior thorax–18%
   ○ Right arm–9%
   ○ Left arm–9%
   ○ Perineum–1%
   ○ Right leg–18%
   ○ Left leg 18%
	❏ For proper treatment and cure

❏ First aid management of burns patient is: Cool, cover and call	❏ Cool all burns with tepid to cool water regardless of degree of burns. Continue flushing the area up to 10 minutes. Remove all clothings or garments to reduce contact. ❏ Cover affected area with a clean dry cloth, towel or blanket to protect the burn and minimize pain. ❏ Seek medical attention if burn is larger than the victims hand size.
❏ Cover the patient with sterile sheet	Sterility protects from risk of infection
❏ Monitor urine output	To maintain fluid balance in the body

Initial Care of Patient in the Burn Unit

NOTES

CHAPTER 56

Fluid Replacement in Acute Burns

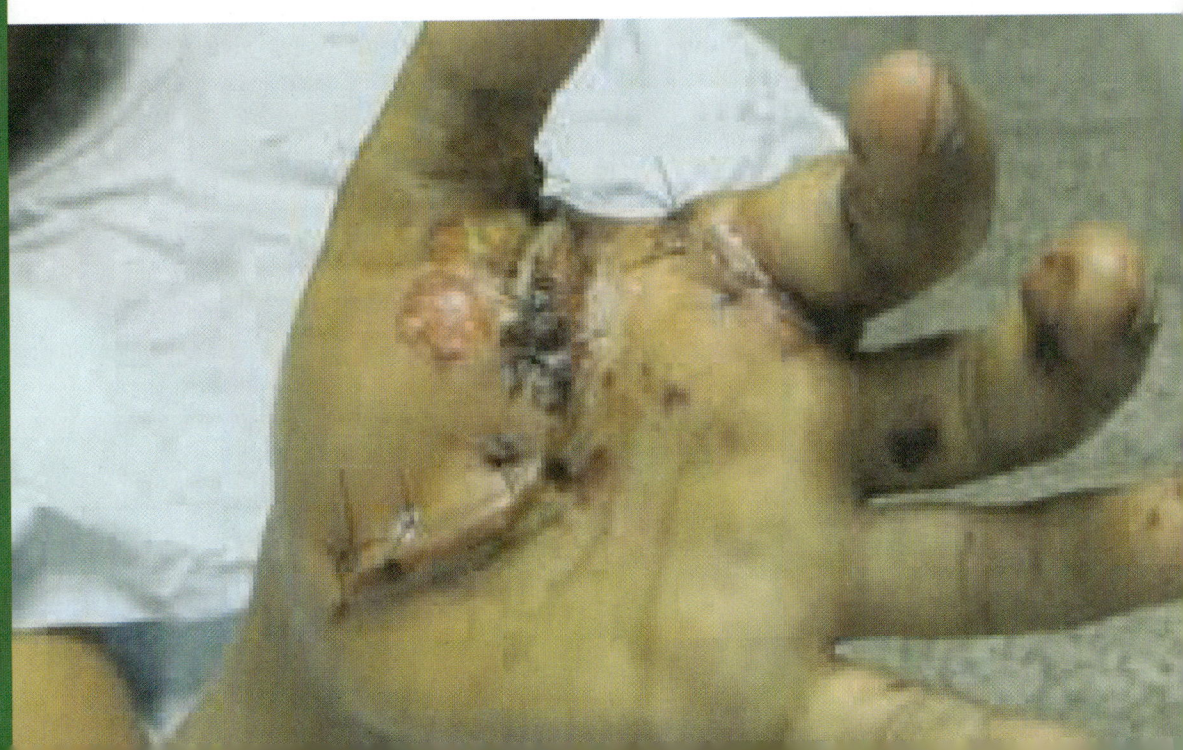

DEFINITION

Fluid resuscitation in burns is to provide and maintain fluid balance.

PURPOSES

- ❑ To prevent complications of burn
- ❑ To prevent hypovolemic shock

INDICATION

- ❑ Patient with burns.

ARTICLES REQUIRED AND THEIR PURPOSES

Articles	Purposes
❑ Cut down set—Sterile pack	❑ To remove the slough over the burns area
❑ Injection xylocaine 2%	❑ To reduce the pain
❑ Disposable needle and syringe	❑ To aspirate the fluid
❑ Scalpel blade no. 11	❑ To administer fluid from other way
❑ 3-way connector	❑ To replace the fluid
❑ Cavafix and transparent tape	
❑ Intravenous (IV) fluid as required	

STEPS OF PROCEDURE AND RATIONALE

Steps	Rationale
❑ Collect information regarding date and time of burn	❑ Help in fluid calculation
❑ Explain procedure to the patient	❑ Help in obtaining cooperation of the patient
❑ Check the weight of the patient	❑ Helps in determining the amount of fluid to be infused
❑ Assist for cut down and connect IV fluids as per order for maintaining fluid balance	❑ Maintain homeostasis
❑ Collect blood samples while cut down	❑ For investigating electrolyte, hematocrit, grouping cross matching and HIV etc.
❑ Monitor urinary output	❑ To understand fluid balance
❑ Check vital signs of the patient	
❑ Continuous cardiac monitoring of the patient	❑ To recognize any changes in normal functioning of heart
❑ Perform hand hygiene	❑ To prevent cross infection
❑ Discard the waste, clean and replace the articles	❑ Keep ready for next use
❑ Record on nurse's notes	

Points to Remember

- ❑ Assess the adequacy of fluid by use of more than one parameters (urine output, blood pressure, etc.)
- ❑ While doing calculation for fluid resuscitation consider the time of burns.

CHAPTER 57

Range of Motion

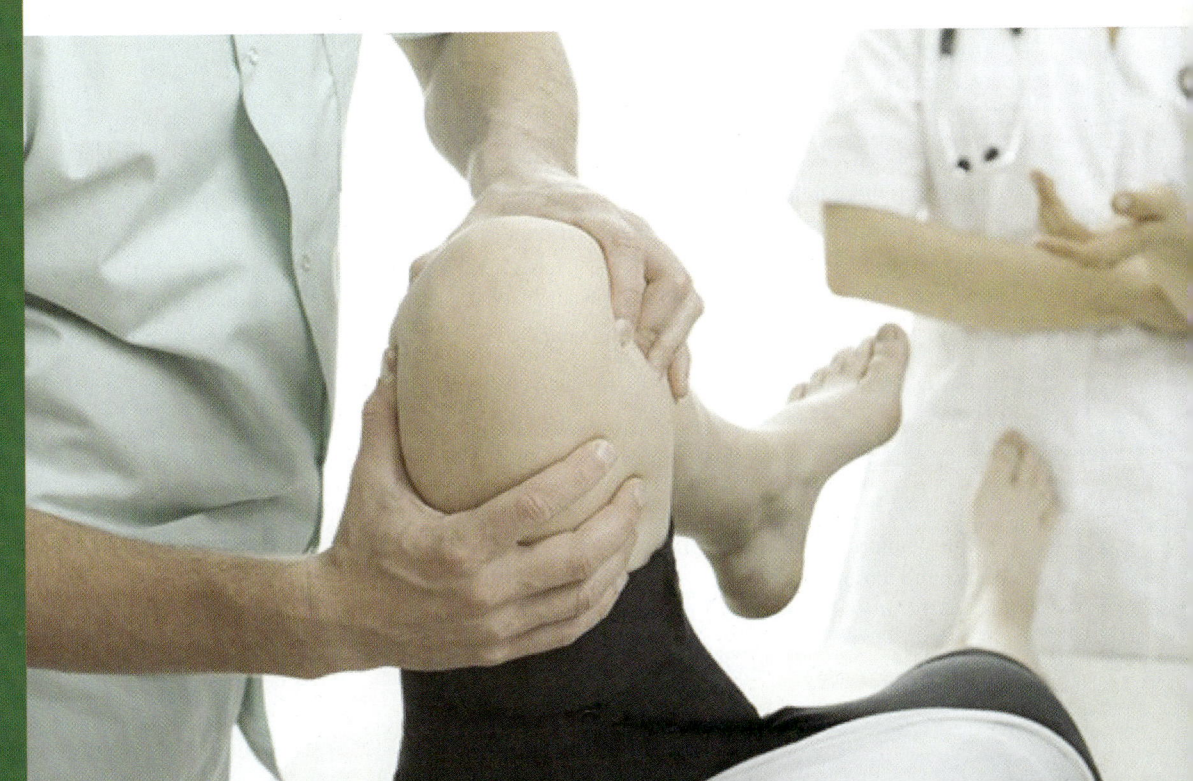

DEFINITION

Range of motion exercise helps to prevent contractures and stiffness of joint by movement of all joints.

PURPOSES

- ❑ To restore normal motion of joints
- ❑ To restore coordination of all the joints
- ❑ To prevent contractures
- ❑ To promote comfort
- ❑ To improve circulation

TYPES OF RANGE OF MOTION

- ❑ **Passive:** Patient need assistance.
- ❑ **Active:** Patient can perform exercise without assistance.
- ❑ **Active assistive:** Patient need very little assistance.

PRELIMINARY ASSESSMENT

Preparation of the Patient

- ❑ Explain the procedure to the patient
- ❑ Adjust the height of the bed if needed
- ❑ Provide comfortable position to the patient
- ❑ If require raise the side railing

Articles

No instruments or articles required for range of motion exercise.

STEPS OF PROCEDURE AND RATIONALE

Steps	Rationale
❑ Wash hands thoroughly	❑ Prevent cross infection
❑ Support the extremity to be moved above and below joint. Do not hold a joint	❑ For easy movement
❑ Perform all movements smoothly and slowly	❑ To avoid discomfort and pain
❑ Move joints through full range of motion. If patient complaints of pain do not force movement	❑ Pain causes discomfort and restricts movement
❑ Perform each movements 3–5 times during exercise per day	❑ For better effect

AFTER CARE

- ❑ Provide comfortable position to the patient.
- ❑ Wash hand thoroughly.
- ❑ Record the procedure in nurse's notes.

ANNEXURES

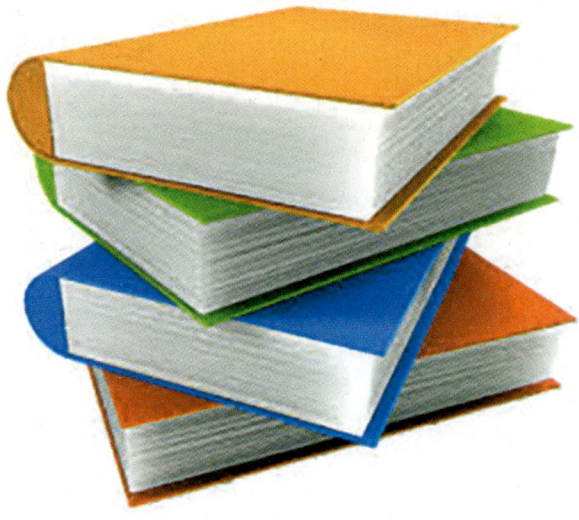

ANNEXURE-I

FLUID CALCULATION CHART

Date	IV fluids	Starting time	Ending time	Calculation	Remark

ANNEXURE-II

HEALTH TALK ASSIGNMENT

Name of Student Teacher: _____

Name of Evaluator: _____

Topic of Health Talk: _____

Group: _____

Date,Time and Venue: _____

Methods of Teaching: _____

Previous Knowledge of Group:

General Objective: _____

Specific Objective: _____

LESSON PLAN

S. No	Specific objective	Time	Content of topic	Teaching-learning activity	AV aids	Evaluation

Summary and Conclusion: Recapitalization:

Bibliography and References:

ANNEXURE-III

MEDICATION CARD

Date	Doctor's order	Ordered dose	Available dose	Route	Time

Student's Signature   Supervisor's Signature

Diet	Special Order

ANNEXURE-IV

BRADEN SCALE FOR PREDICTING PRESSURE SORE RISK

Write score 1-4

		Completely limited	Very limited responds	Slightly limited	No impairment	
A	**Sensory perception** Ability to respond meaningfully to pressure-related discomfort.	**Completely limited** Unresponsive (does not moan, flinch, or grasp) to painful stimuli, due to diminished level of consciousness or sedation or limited ability to feel pain over most of body.	**Very limited responds** only to painful stimuli. Cannot communicate discomfort except by moaning or restlessness **OR** has a sensory impairment which limits the ability to feel pain or discomfort over 2 of body.	**Slightly limited** Responds to verbal commands, but cannot always communicate discomfort or the need to be turned. **OR** has some sensory impairment which limits ability to feel pain or discomfort in 1 or 2 extremities.	**No impairment** Responds to verbal commands. Has no sensory deficit which would limit ability to feel or voice pain or discomfort.	
B	**Moisture** Degree to which skin is exposed to moisture.	**Constantly moist** Skin is kept moist almost constantly by perspiration, urine, etc. Dampness is detected every time patient is moved or turned.	**Very moist** Skin is often, but not always moist. Linen must be changed at least once a shift.	**Occasionally moist** Skin is occasionally moist, requiring an extra linen change approximately once a day.	**Rarely moist** Skin is usually dry, linen only requires changing at routine intervals.	
C	**Activity** Degree of physical activity.	**Bedfast** Confined to bed.	**Chairfast** Ability to walk severely limited or non-existent. Cannot bear own weight and/or must be assisted into chair or wheelchair.	**Walks occasionally** Walks occasionally during day, but for very short distances, with or without assistance. Spends majority of each shift in bed or chair	**Walks frequently** Walks outside room at least twice a day and inside room at least once every two hours during waking hours.	
D	**Mobility** Ability to change and control body position.	**Completely immobile** Does not make even slight changes in body or extremity position without assistance.	**Very limited** Makes occasional slight changes in body or extremity position but unable to make frequent or significant changes independently.	**Slightly limited** Makes frequent though slight changes in body or extremity position independently.	**No limitation** Makes major and frequent changes in position without assistance.	

Contd…

Annexures

E	Nutrition Usual food intake pattern.	Very poor Never eats a complete meal. Rarely eats more than any food offered. Eats 2 servings or less of protein (meat or dairy products) per day. Takes fluids poorly. Does not take a liquid dietary supplement OR is NPO and/or maintained on clear liquids or IVs for more than 5 days.	Probably inadequate Rarely eats a complete meal and generally eats only about 2 of any food offered. Protein intake includes only 3 servings of meat or dairy products per day. Occasionally will take a dietary supplement. OR receives less than optimum amount of liquid diet or tube feeding.	Adequate Eats over half of most meals. Eats a total of 4 servings of protein (meat, dairy products per day. Occasionally will refuse a meal, but will usually take a supplement when offered OR is on a tube feeding or TPN regimen which probably meets most of nutritional needs.	Excellent Eats most of every meal. Never refuses a meal. Usually eats a total of 4 or more servings of meat and dairy products. Occasionally eats between meals. Does not require supplementation.	
F	Friction and shear	Problem Requires moderate to maximum assistance in moving. Complete lifting without sliding against sheets is impossible. Frequently slides down in bed or chair, requiring frequent repositioning with maximum assistance. Spasticity, contractures or agitation leads to almost constant friction.	Potential problem Moves feebly or requires minimum assistance. During a move skin probably slides to some extent against sheets, chair, restraints or other devices. Maintains relatively good position in chair or bed most of the time but occasionally slides down.	No apparent problem Moves in bed and in chair independently and has sufficient muscle strength to lift up completely during move. Maintains good position in bed or chair.		

A + B + C + D + E + F = Total score:

Pressure sore risk	
Xtra high risk:	= 9 Points
High risk:	= 10-12 Points
Medium risk:	= 13-14 Points
Low risk:	= 15-16 Points

Patient's Name:_____ Evaluator's Name: _____ Date:_____

VIP Score Visual Infusion Phlebitis Score (VIP Score)

IV site appears healthy	0	No sign of phlebitis ❑ Observe cannula
One of the following is evident: ❑ Slight pain near the IV ❑ Site or slight redness near the IV site	1	Possible first sign of phlebitis ❑ Observe cannula
Two of the following are evident: ❑ Pale near IV site ❑ Erythema ❑ Swelling	2	Early stage of phlebitis ❑ Resite cannula
All of the following are evident: ❑ Pain along path of cannula ❑ Erythema ❑ Induration	3	Medium stage of phlebitis ❑ Resite cannula ❑ Consider treatment
All of the following are evident and extensive: ❑ Pain along path of cannula ❑ Erythema ❑ Induration ❑ Palpable venous cord	4	Advanced stage of phlebitis or start of thrombophlebitis ❑ Resite cannula ❑ Consider treatment
All of the following are evident and extensive: ❑ Pain along path of cannula ❑ Erythema ❑ Induration ❑ Palpable venous cord ❑ **Pyrexia**	5	Advanced stage of thrombophlebitis ❑ Initiate treatment ❑ Resite cannula

NOTES

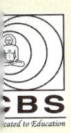
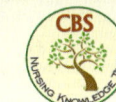

First Book on Nursing Procedures Developed by the Most Renowned Institute NINE-PGIMER
Covers more than 250 Procedures in all Nursing Subjects; Edited by the Leading Subject Experts of the Institute

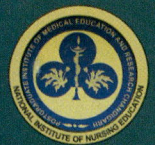
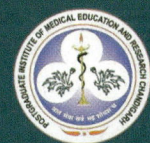

Postgraduate Institute of Medical Education & Research (PGIMER), Chandigarh
National Institute of Nursing Education (NINE)

CLINICAL NURSING PROCEDURES

- *Nursing Foundations*
- *Medical Surgical Nursing*
- *Mental Health Nursing*
- *Obstetric & Gynecological Nursing*
- *Pediatric Nursing*
- *Community Health Nursing*

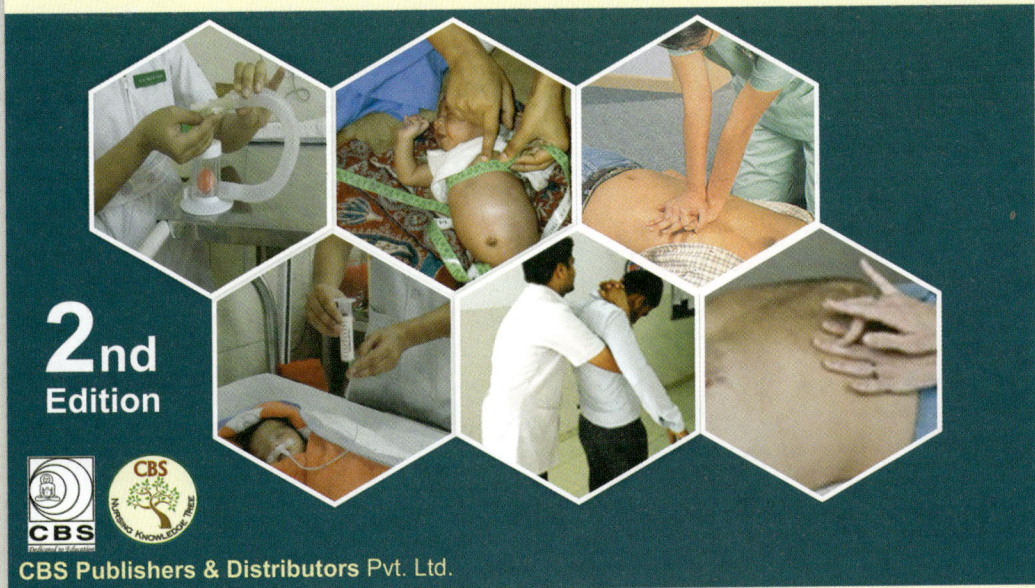

2nd Edition

CBS

CBS Publishers & Distributors Pvt. Ltd.

Forewords
Jagat Ram
Subhash Varma
Anil Kumar Gupta

Editor-in-Chief
Sandhya Ghai

Editors
- Avinash Kaur Rana
- Sunita Sharma
- Sushma Kumari Saini
- Sukhpal Kaur
- Sukhwinder Kaur
- Neena Vir Singh

ISBN: 978-93-86478-93-1
Pages: 1200

2/e, 2019
MRP ₹1250/-

CBS Publishers & Distributors Pvt. Ltd.
• New Delhi • Bengaluru • Chennai • Kochi • Kolkata • Mumbai • Pune • Hyderabad • Nagpur • Patna • Vijayawada

Above books available at **All Medical Book Stores of India**
For any availability issue please contact : +91-9555590180

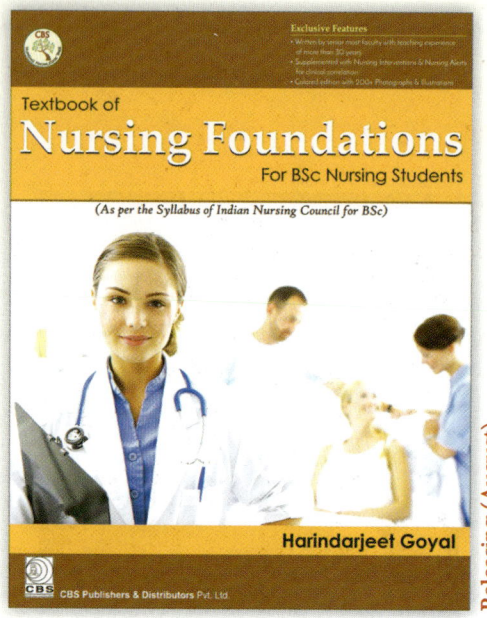

Textbook of Nursing Foundations For BSc Nursing Students

Harindarjeet Goyal

Releasing (August)

ISBN: 978-93-88108-94-2
Pages: 800 (T)
1/e, 2019
MRP *TBA

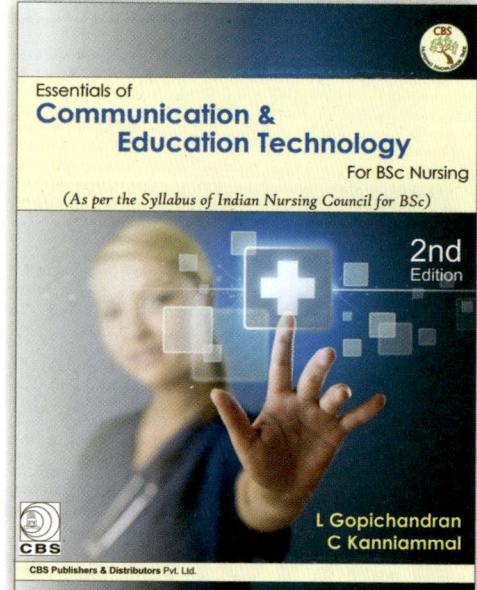

Essentials of Communication & Education Technology For BSc Nursing

L Gopichandran
C Kanniammal

ISBN: 978-93-88178-58-7
Pages: 336
2/e, 2019
MRP ₹450/-

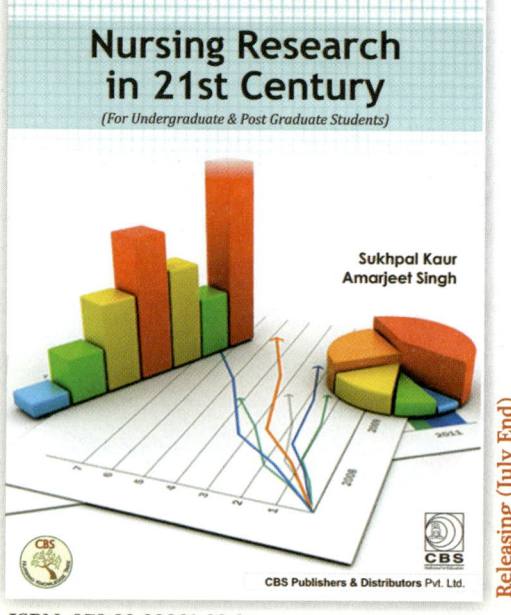

Nursing Research in 21st Century (For Undergraduate & Post Graduate Students)

Sukhpal Kaur
Amarjeet Singh

Releasing (July End)

ISBN: 978-93-89261-89-9
Pages: 1000 (T)
1/e, 2019
MRP *TBA

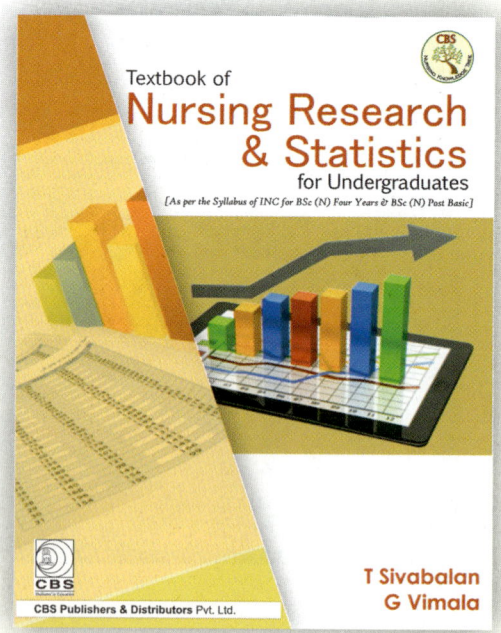

Textbook of Nursing Research & Statistics for Undergraduates

T Sivabalan
G Vimala

ISBN: 978-93-88178-61-7
Pages: 290
1/e, 2018
MRP ₹495/-

 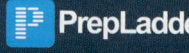 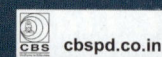 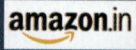 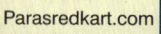 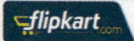 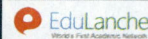

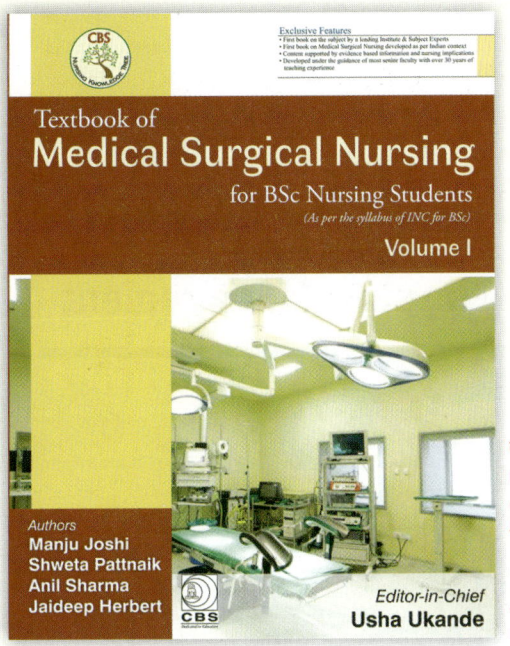

ISBN: 978-93-88178-54-9

Pages: 1000 (T)

1/e, 2019

MRP *TBA

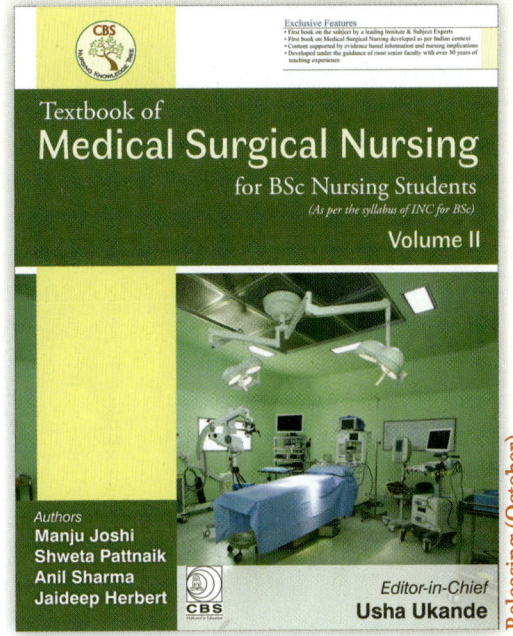

Pages: 800 (T)

1/e, 2019

MRP *TBA

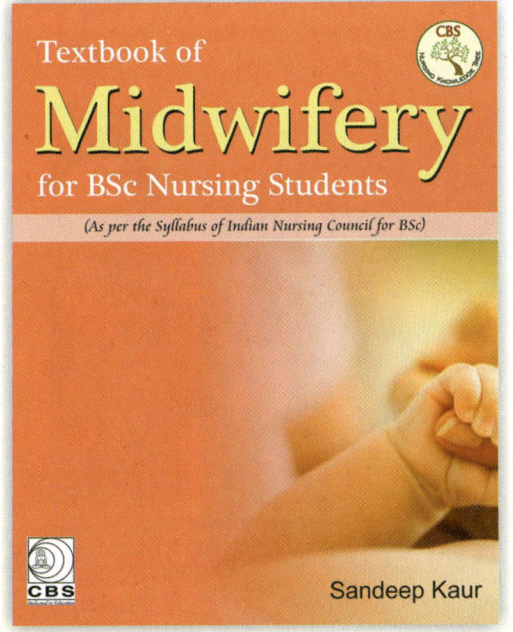

ISBN: 978-93-89261-90-5

Pages: 450 (T)

1/e, 2019

MRP *TBA

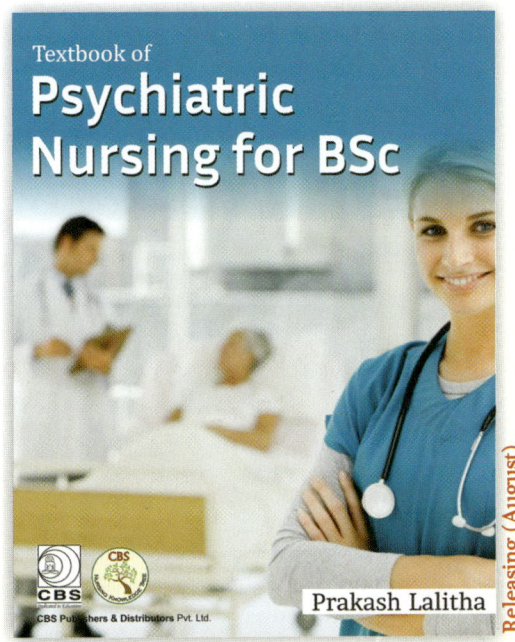

ISBN: 978-93-89261-91-2

Pages: 500 (T)

1/e, 2019

MRP *TBA

CBS Publishers & Distributors Pvt. Ltd.

• New Delhi • Bengaluru • Chennai • Kochi • Kolkata • Mumbai • Pune • Hyderabad • Nagpur • Patna • Vijayawada

Above books available at **All Medical Book Stores of India**

For any availability issue please contact : +91-9555590180

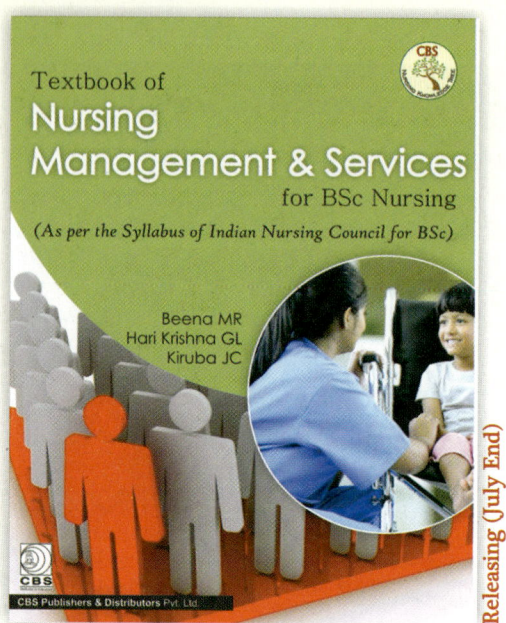

Releasing (July End)

ISBN: 978-93-88178-62-4
Pages: 500 (T)

1/e, 2019
MRP *TBA

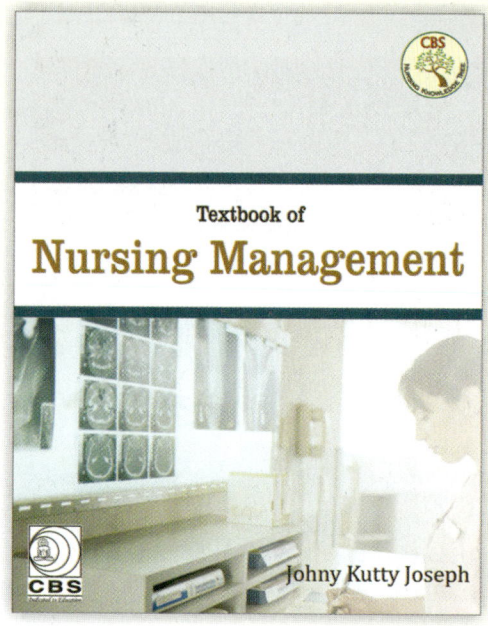

Releasing (August)

Pages: 450 (T)

1/e, 2019
MRP *TBA

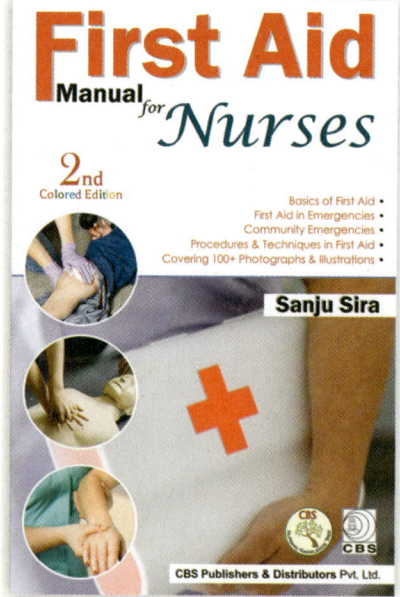

ISBN: 978-93-88178-55-6
Pages: 208

2/e, 2019
MRP ₹295/-

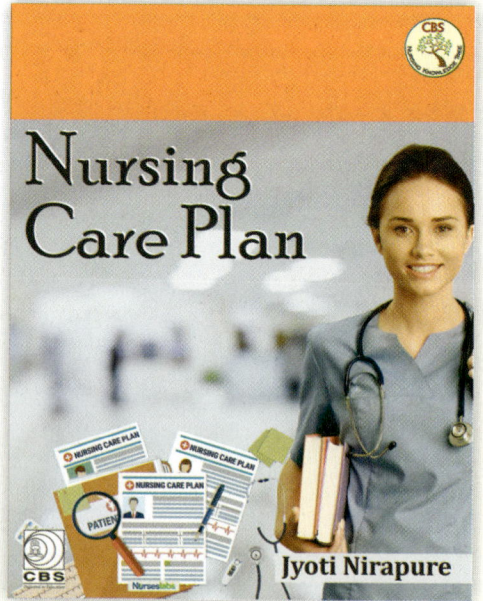

Releasing (July End)

ISBN: 978-93-89261-96-7
Pages: 250 (T)

1/e, 2019
MRP *TBA

 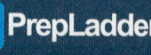 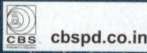 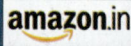 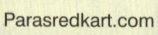 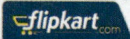 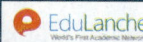

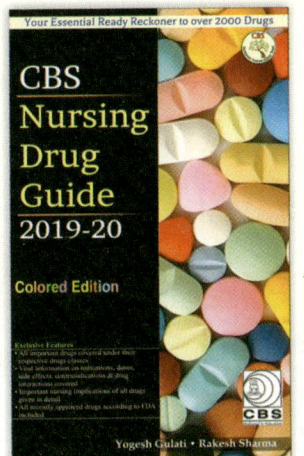

Releasing (August)

ISBN: 978-93-88178-52-5
Pages: 800 (T)
1/e, 2019
MRP *TBA

Releasing (August)

ISBN: 978-93-88178-53-2
Pages: 800 (T)
1/e, 2019
MRP *TBA

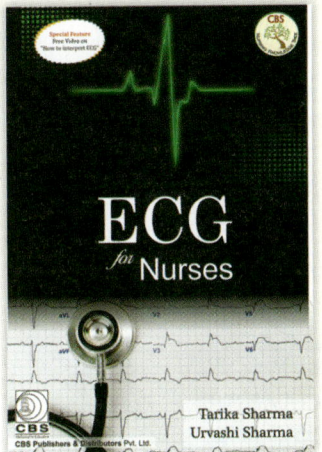

Releasing (July End)

ISBN: 978-93-89261-88-2
Pages: 200 (T)
1/e, 2019
MRP *TBA

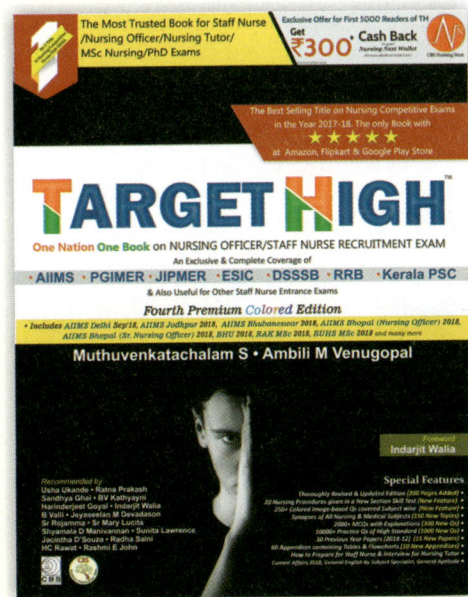

ISBN: 978-93-87964-78-5   4/e, 2018-19
Pages: 1232   MRP ₹1199/-

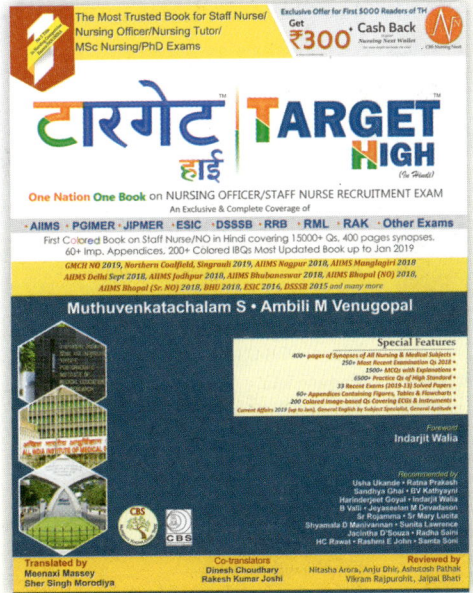

ISBN: 978-93-88178-63-1   1/e, 2019
Pages: 1300   MRP ₹1099/-

CBS Publishers & Distributors Pvt. Ltd.

• New Delhi • Bengaluru • Chennai • Kochi • Kolkata • Mumbai • Pune • Hyderabad • Nagpur • Patna • Vijayawada

Above books available at **All Medical Book Stores of India**
For any availability issue please contact : +91-9555590180

Nursing Textbooks (B.Sc)

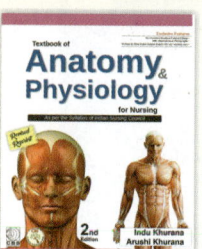

Textbook of
Anatomy & Physiology
for Nursing
Indu Khurana & Arushi Khurana

ISBN: 978-93-86827-12-8
Pages: 568
2/e, 2018 (Revised Reprint)
MRP ₹950/-

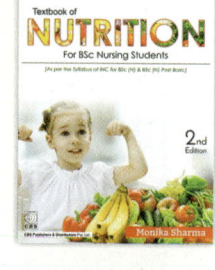

Textbook of
Nutrition
for BSc Nursing Students
Monika Sharma

ISBN: 978-93-89261-92-9
Pages: 300
2/e, 2019
MRP ₹350/- (T)

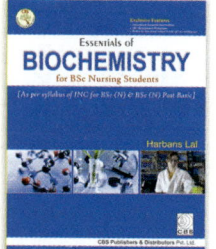

Essentials of
Biochemistry
for BSc Nursing Students
Harbans Lal

ISBN: 978-81-23927-19-0
Pages: 332
1/e, 2017-18
MRP ₹425/-

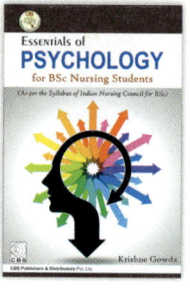

Essentials of ### Psychology
for BSc Nursing Students
Krishne Gowda

ISBN: 978-81-23927-11-4
Pages: 362
1/e, 2017-18
MRP ₹325/-

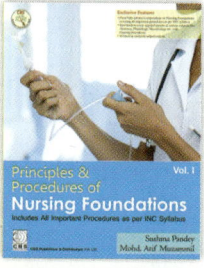

Principles & Procedures of Nursing Foundations (Vol. I)
(Basic Procedures)
Sushma Pandey & Mohd. Atif Muzammil

ISBN: 978-93-88108-95-9
Pages: 392
1/e, 2019
MRP ₹595/- (T)

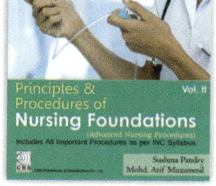

Principles & Procedures of Nursing Foundations (Vol.
(Advanced Nursing Procedures)
Sushma Pandey & Mohd. Atif Muzam.

ISBN: 978-93-89261-87-5
Pages: 300 (T)
1/e, 2019
MRP ₹395/- (T)

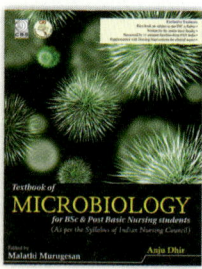

Textbook of
Microbiology for
BSc & Post Basic Nursing Students
Anju Dhir

ISBN: 978-93-88108-82-9
Pages: 535
1/e, 2018-19
MRP ₹695/-

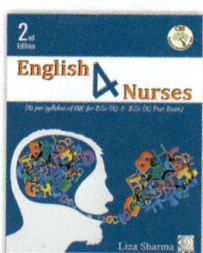

English 4 Nurses
for BSc
Liza Sharma

ISBN: 978-93-89261-95-0
Pages: 450
2/e, 2019
MRP ₹395/- (T)

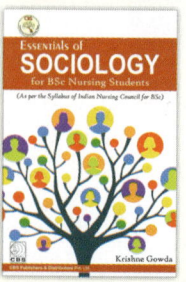

Essentials of
Sociology for
BSc Nusing Students
Krishne Gowda

ISBN: 978-93-86217-51-6
Pages: 362
1/e, 2017
MRP ₹375/-

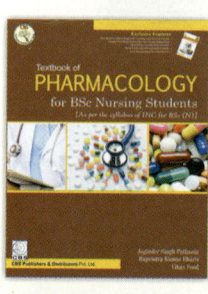

Textbook of ### Pharmacology
for BSc Nursing Students
Joginder Singh Pathania
Rupendra Kr. Bharti
Vikas Sood

ISBN: 978-93-86217-80-6
Pages: 486
1/e, 2017-18
MRP ₹595/-

  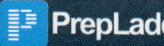 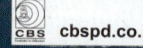 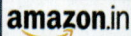 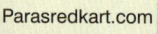 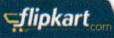 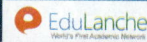

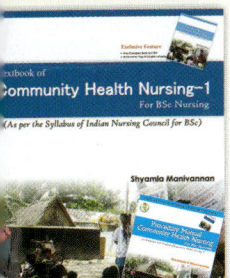

Textbook of
Community Health Nursing-I for BSc Nursing
Shyamala D Manivannan

ISBN: 978-81-23927-01-5
Pages: 508
1/e, 2018
MRP ₹725/-

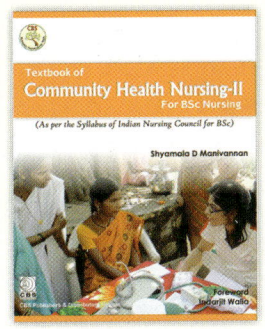

Textbook of
Community Health Nursing-II for BSc Nursing
Shyamala D Manivannan

ISBN: 978-93-86827-22-7
Pages: 326
1/e, 2018
MRP ₹425/-

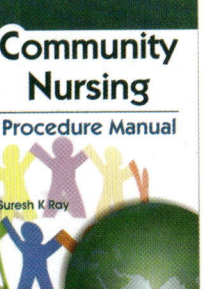

Community Nursing
Procedure Manual
Suresh K Ray

ISBN: 978-81-23929-35-4
Pages: 179
1/e, 2017
MRP ₹250/-

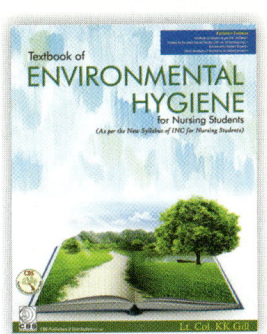

Textbook of
Environmental Hygiene
for Nursing Students
Lt. Col. KK Gill

ISBN: 978-93-88178-56-3
Pages: 110
1/e, 2018-19
MRP ₹195/-

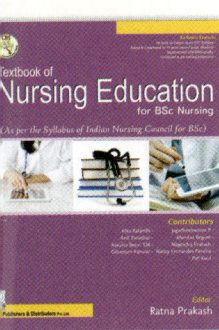

Textbook of
Nursing Education
for BSc Nursing
Ratna Prakash

ISBN: 978-93-86827-34-0
Pages: 340
1/e, 2018
MRP ₹425/-

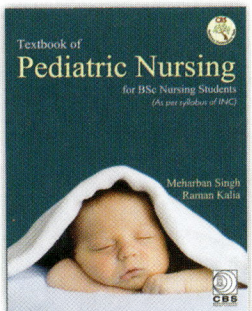

Textbook of
Pediatric Nursing
for BSc Nursing Students
Meharban Singh & Raman Kalia

ISBN: 978-93-88108-72-0
Pages: 630
1/e, 2018-19
MRP ₹695/-

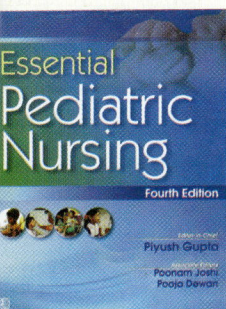

Essential
Pediatric Nursing
Piyush Gupta

ISBN: 978-93-86217-87-5
Pages: 576
4/e, 2017
MRP ₹725/-

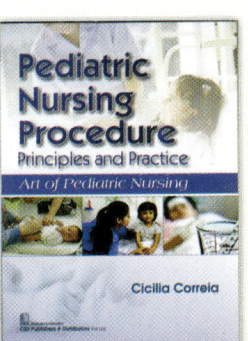

Pediatric Nursing Procedure Principles and Practice
Art of Pediatric Nursing
Cicilia Correia

ISBN: 978-93-86310-74-3
Pages: 360
1/e, 2017
MRP ₹425/-

CBS Publishers & Distributors Pvt. Ltd.
• New Delhi • Bengaluru • Chennai • Kochi • Kolkata • Mumbai • Pune • Hyderabad • Nagpur • Patna • Vijayawada

Above books available at **All Medical Book Stores of India**
For any availability issue please contact : +91-9555590180

Nursing Textbooks for B.Sc

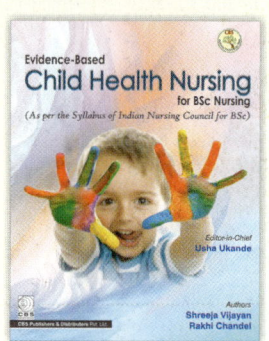

Evidence-Based
Child Health Nursing
for BSc Nursing
Usha Ukande

Pages: 800 (T)
1/e, 2019
Releasing Soon

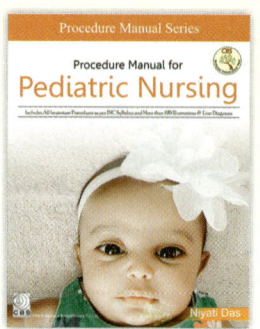

Procedure Manual for
Pediatric Nursing
Niyati Das

ISBN: 978-93-88108-86-7
Pages: 235
1/e, 2018-19
MRP ₹295/-

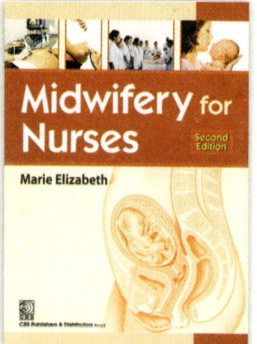

Midwifery for Nurses
Marie Elizabeth

ISBN: 978-81-23922-14-0
Pages: 544
2/e, 2018-19
MRP ₹625/-

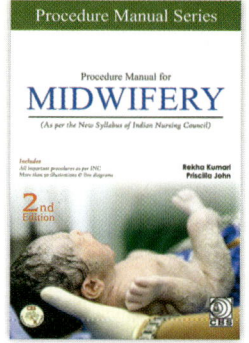

Procedure Manual for
Midwifery
Rekha Kumari & Priscilla John

ISBN: 978-93-89261-94-3
Pages: 200 (T)
2/e, 2019
Releasing (July End)

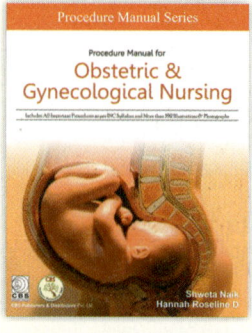

Procedure Manual for ## Obstetric & Gynecological Nursing
Shweta Naik & Hannah Roseline D

ISBN: 978-93-88178-60-0
Pages: 200
1/e, 2018-19
MRP ₹225/-

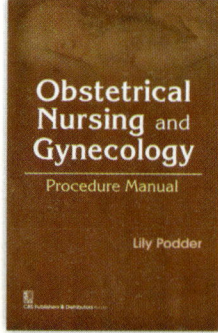

Obstetrical Nursing and Gynecology
Procedure Manual
Lily Podder

ISBN: 978-81-23925-81-3
Pages: 116
1/e, 2017
MRP ₹250/-

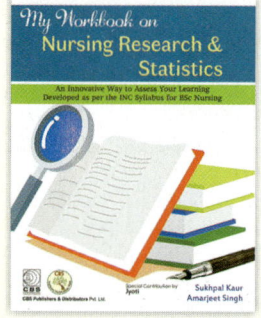

My Workbook on
Nursing Res. & Statistics
Sukhpal Kaur & Amarjeet Singh

ISBN: 978-93-88108-75-1
Pages: 80
1/e, 2019
MRP ₹125/-

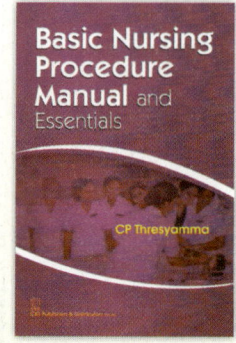

Basic Nursing Procedure Manual and Essentials
CP Thresyamma

ISBN: 978-81-23924-29-8
Pages: 648
1/e, 2017
MRP ₹495/-

 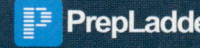 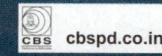 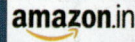 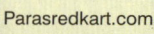 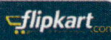 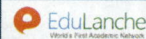